Fibromyalgia Relief

THE SAM-e SOLUTION

Fibromyalgia Relief

THE SAM-e SOLUTION

≈

*Including a Comprehensive Guide
to Other Drug-free Self-care Remedies*

≈

Joseph K. Egbebike, PhD, PT

.

PTS PUBLISHING COMPANY
OLD BRIDGE, NEW JERSEY

Fibromyalgia Relief: The SAM-e Solution
Including a Comprehensive Guide to Other Drug-free Self-care Remedies
Copyright ©2000 by Joseph K. Egbebike

ISBN 0-9639841-2-8

Library of Congress Control Number: 00-090461

PTS Publishing Company • P.O. Box 663 • Old Bridge, NJ 08857
732-296-1111 • www.ptspublishing.com

Publisher's Cataloging-in-Publication
(Provided by Quality Books, Inc.)
Egbebike, Joseph K.
   Fibromyalgia relief : the SAM-e solution,
   including a comprehensive guide to other drug-free
   self-care remedies / by Joseph K. Egbebike, -- 1st
   ed.
      p. cm.
      LCCN: 00-090461
      ISBN: 0-9639841-2-8

      1. Fibromyalgia--Alternative treatment.
   2. Adenosylmethionine--Therapeutic use.   1. Title.

RC927.3.E44 2000   616.7'4
                                QBI00-242

Cover design by Dunn & Associates
Interior book design by Sue Knopf/Graffolio
Illustrations by Bob Calleja

Contents

Part 1: Overview of Fibromyalgia Syndrome

*So what is this thing called fibromyalgia? • Who gets
fibromyalgia? • Children and fibromyalgia • Economic
cost of fibromyalgia • Can fibromyalgia be inherited? •
Who is at risk? • How does fibromyalgia progress?*

*Chronic fatigue syndrome • Lyme disease • Lupus
Polymyalgia Rheumatica (PMR) • Rheumatoid diseases
• Sjögren's Syndrome • Common symptoms of
fibromyalgia and associated disorders*

*Uniqueness of fibromyalgia • American College of
Rheumatology's 1990 criteria*

*Hereditary factors • Chronic sleep disorder • Abnormal
brain function • Autoimmune disorder • Post-traumatic
stress disorder • Trauma • Muscle cell abnormality •
Low levels of Vitamin B_{12} and high levels of homocysteine
in CSF • Viral infection*

*Drugs for sleep disorders, fatigue, irritable bowel syn-
drome and headaches • Modes of action of common
drugs used to treat fibromyalgia*

Part 2: Re-evaluating Your Medications

Part 3: SAM-e to the Rescue

SAM-e and gene expression abnormality • SAM-e and sleep disorders • SAM-e, abnormal brain function and neurotransmitter regulation • SAM-e and high CSF homocysteine levels • SAM-e and autoimmune disorder • SAM-e and depressive moods and fatigue • SAM-e, muscle pain and tender points • SAM-e and migraine headaches • SAM-e's role in controlling system levels of toxins, oxidants, histamine and allergens • Recent scientific studies on the effects of SAM-e on fibromyalgia.

Part 4: Other Drug-Free Fibromyalgia Relief and Self-care Strategies

Part 5: Fibromyalgia Disability Issues and Conclusions

List of Illustrations

Author's Biography

Joseph K. Egbebike, Ph.D., PT, is the Executive Director of Comprehensive Healthcare Center, a medical rehabilitation and pain relief facility with offices in Somerset and Holmdel, New Jersey.

Dr. Egbebike holds a doctorate in Pathokinesiology from New York University. He has been a licensed physical therapist and pain relief specialist for more than 17 years. He has also set up and managed rehabilitation programs at several healthcare centers in New Jersey, Michigan, Ohio and Vermont. He is board-certified in three states. He is a member of the American Physical Therapy Association, American College of Sports Medicine, and American Congress of Rehabilitation, among others.

Comprehensive Healthcare Centers specialize in the treatment of fibromyalgia and chronic pain, using integrative, holistic and multidisciplinary methods, and have been offering free educational lectures to the public on the subject.

Other publications by the author include:

Complying with O.B.R.A.: Managing Restraint Reduction Programs in Nursing Homes and Healthcare Centers, ISBN: 0-9639841-0-1 (Published 1993)

Introduction

Surprisingly, there are some nice things that can be said about pain. Experiencing pain goes hand in hand with the phenomenon of Life. We are able to feel pain because we are alive. In fact, we learn to live more fully after we have survived pain and suffering. It is our common human heritage. No one can avoid it, no matter how powerful or rich one is. Pain in one form or the other will find and grip each of us from time to time.

But as unpleasant as it is, the experience of enduring pain has a positive side. The fact is, pain teaches us much more about ourselves than any other thing could. We learn to appreciate what we have, while developing more empathy for those who are less fortunate than we are. So pain now and then is always normal. But constant pain, the kind that makes you feel as if you have a perpetual flu, is not normal. It is this kind of abnormal experience with pain that Christine has experienced.

Christine's problems started about eight years ago. She sustained a whiplash injury after a drunken motorist slammed into the back of her stopped car as she waited at a red light. Since then her symptoms have multiplied and become more intense. She is only thirty-eight years old, but she now feels as though she is sixty. She has been forced to quit her job as a schoolteacher. To make matters worse, she has been unable to obtain disability assistance, despite her efforts to do so since the accident.

Before her accident, in spite of her childhood diagnosis of scoliosis, she had developed and maintained an active, sports-oriented lifestyle since seventh grade. But since the accident, everything has changed. Outwardly, Christine looks fine, but inwardly, she feels terrible. Constant pain with fatigue and sleepless nights rob her body's natural energy. She had run the gamut of doctors and therapists; taken countless MRIs, X-rays, CAT scans and blood work-ups. But then, three years ago, one of those doctors had the good sense to refer her to a rheumatologist.

Dr. Kane was sympathetic and kind. He seemed to know a lot about her condition. It wasn't long before he put a name on her disease and diagnosed her with fibromyalgia. In Dr. Kane's view, the whiplash injury may have been the precipitating factor. Ordinarily, he said, there is no certain cause for fibromyalgia or any complete cure. Of the thirteen so-called tender points tested on Christine, eleven were very painful on palpation.

He prescribed a daily dose of 25 mg of Amitryptyline to be taken with up to 400 mg of Ibuprofen at night to help her sleep problems. She feels better some days, while the pain is more intense on other days. To complicate matters, she was unable to participate in the physical therapy program to which her doctor had referred her to help ease the pain because the pain was already too overwhelming.

Christine has needed to increase her dosages and has gradually developed other problems, such as dizziness, diarrhea, nausea and vomiting. She also gained weight and developed symptoms of depression. Efforts to decrease her dosage-or even stop completely-resulted in a worsening of some of her symptoms. Andy, her husband of nine years, who has been supportive in the past, has grown weary of the ups and downs and become irritable with her.

The fact is, Christine's story is not at all unique. Most of the participants at the public free lectures our practice (Comprehensive Healthcare) gives complain of the same things. Most of them are on one form or another of tricyclic antidepressant. Prescribing these medications is standard practice, yet they often cause serious side effects that greatly affect patients' lifestyles.

Fibromyalgia is unique to rheumatic type diseases in its failure to express itself in an objective set of symptoms, such as active inflammations, or the showing of positive results in lab work. Its genesis is only conjecture, and treatment that is purely empirical. Doctors use the same medications for the treatment of fibromyalgia that they use for their arthritis patients. As yet, there are no FDA-approved drugs for fibromyalgia, so there are no clear guidelines about dosages or drug interaction. Furthermore, there seems to be some consensus among researchers that fibromyalgia is not in fact a psychiatric condition. Rather, depression is often a resulting condition arising from the frustration of attempting to manage productive life while enduring a debilitating disease that has no cure in sight.

In fact, the medications may be adding to the problem. According to internationally famous psychiatrist, Peter R. Breggin, M.D., author of *Talking Back to Prozac* and *Toxic Psychiatry*, the human brain is more complex and mysterious than the entire Universe. Medicine, besides not being an exact science, has not even begun to unravel the mysteries of the brain-the intricacies of its internal structures—nor the zillion interconnections between its cells or numerous chemical messengers, known as neurotransmitters, whose functions modern science barely understands.

According to Drs. Breggin and Cohen, in their book *Your Drug May be Your Problem,* "The knowledge that we have about the effects of psychiatric drugs on the brain is largely limited to test tube studies of biochemical reactions utilizing ground-up pieces of animal brain. We simply do not understand the overall impact of drugs on the brain."

Personally, I have always believed that too much dependence on medications-especially psychiatric ones-robs us of our natural spontaneity to life's dilemmas. On psychiatric medications, we disconnect from our inner minds and natural self-healing potential. I think many clinicians are too quick to prescribe antidepressants and antibiotics without discussing other non-pharmacological options with their patients. A 15-minute decision by the doctor may change a patient's life forever. Most of the research studies on which their decisions are based are really nothing but well-funded propaganda by the ultra-wealthy drug companies. If there were a way clinicians could try out these drugs themselves, I am certain that they would become less enthusiastic about prescribing them for their patients.

It is therefore with great excitement that I learned about SAM-e. Since then, I have read whatever I could lay my hands on regarding the subject. SAM-e (pronounced Sammy) was only recently approved for US markets. But SAM-e has been used for decades by doctors in Europe with excellent results. Evidence from several scientific studies suggests that SAM-e might be a good substitute for the tricyclic antidepressants currently used to treat fibromyalgia.

In one study, reported in the *Scandinavian Journal of Rheumatology,* 800 mg of SAM-e, taken daily for a period of 6 weeks, was shown to improve patients' "disease activity," relieve pain, morning stiffness and depressive moods. This is in agreement with several other studies we shall discuss in detail later. SAM-e was shown by these studies to work as well as, and even faster than, conventional antidepressants. Most importantly, it does so without the debilitating side effects of the antidepressants.

The field of alternative, or complementary, or integrative medicine has recently gained momentum. A recent study in the *Journal of American Medical Association* reported that Americans spend about 27 billion dollars yearly on alternative medicine, herbs, and books on the subject. "People don't look for alternatives if they're satisfied with what they've got," says Jack Daniel of the Center for traditional Acupuncture in Columbia, Maryland. People are beginning to realize that they are comprised of more than simply their physical bodies. People are recognizing that in addition to the body, we each have a mind and a soul. They realize that an interconnection and interdependence exist between all of these substrates that make up one person. And with the information superhighway explosion called the Internet, people are now reading the same materials available to their doctors and forming their own opinions about their illnesses and treatment priorities.

Of course, we are all wary of hype, especially in an unregulated supplement like SAM-e. So many unethical players may join the band for a quick profit and the consumer becomes exposed to possible harm. But I do think SAM-e is the way to go for a fibromyalgia relief, at least as a complimentary remedy. My simple argument for SAM-e is this: For a multi-symptomatic chronic condition like fibromyalgia, with no known cause or established pattern of progression, with only a trial and error treatment method available, I think SAM-e is the best choice. Remember that SAM-e is a supplement with no known adverse effects, naturally occurs in the body, and is more involved in the body's self-healing metabolic processes than any other substance in the body except adenosine triphosphate, known as ATP.

It is important to note, though, that neither SAM-e, nor any other supplement nor even drugs, can arrest the problems of fibromyalgia, without the assistance of other self-help strategies. We are supposed to be in charge of our bodies. We need to look into our own inner self-healing resources and coping potentials. We need to address issues of stress and tension in our relationships, knowing that the happiness we give is the very same happiness that we receive.

The chapters of this book have been arranged in a logical sequence and are meant to flow into successive chapters. My main aim in writing this book is to empower you to heal yourself and to be less chemically dependent. It is my fervent hope that after reading it, you will have learned the following:

- the basic facts about SAM-e and fibromyalgia so you can contribute intelligently to your doctor's healthcare decisions, and perhaps try out SAM-e;
- the side effects and withdrawal symptoms of your current medications;
- how to safely come off of your addictive medications;
- correct dosage for SAM-e and how to buy only the right brand;
- several other self-help strategies for stress and muscle soreness, fatigue, sleep problems, etc.;
- appropriate nutritional supplements for fibromyalgia;
- to follow a fibromyalgia-specific fitness and exercise program;
- that you may be eligible for government disability payments if you are out of your job for over a year. The Social Security Administration routinely denies fibromyalgia disability claims for want of objective data on symptoms. Find out how to resolve this problem with the Fibromyalgia Impact Questionnaire.

PART 1

Overview of Fibromyalgia Syndrome

CHAPTER 1

~

Understanding
Fibromyalgia Syndrome (FMS)

The most frequent complaint of fibromyalgia sufferers is that everywhere, everything hurts. Pain is brought on by weather conditions, cold water or even the cold draft rushing in through an open window.

In Christine's case, pain starts from the neck and radiates down the arms and back. Instead of feeling refreshed when she wakes up in the morning, she is still very tired.

In Debbie's case, it was a headache that didn't seem to respond to anything. How frustrating to experience real pain that relatives—even physicians—don't understand. You sometimes have the feeling that they may all be thinking you are imagining it. Other fibromyalgia sufferers have described symptoms akin to those of a perpetual flu and muscle soreness.

So What Is This Thing Called Fibromyalgia?

Prior to the 1990 American College of Rheumatology's definition, there had been some controversy about what the affliction actually was. Some had called it "fibrositis," which of course meant an inflammatory process in the fibrous connective tissues. But soon that term was considered a misnomer, since muscle biopsy reports do not indicate any inflammatory activity. Eventually, a consensus was reached by the American College of Rheumatology, in which the phenomenon was named "fibromyalgia." The word "syndrome" was added to denote its multi-symptomatic nature.

3

According to the College's criteria, fibromyalgia syndrome (FMS) was defined as a chronic disorder characterized by persistent and widespread muscle soreness, stiffness, chronic fatigue and many other symptoms, markedly including well-defined painful spots called "tender points."

Other problems of FMS include problems with concentration or memory difficulty called "fibro-fog." X-rays, CAT scans and blood analyses do not show abnormalities. Most often, sufferers are asked to take things easy, do more exercise and generally try not to mind it. As time goes on and the complaints continue, family support may waver. The spouse gets more irritable as the condition forces lifestyle changes. Many fibromyalgia sufferers develop depressive moods, as the problem seems to take over their lives. They become less active and sociable, hoping to resume their lives as soon as things get better. But it doesn't get better and they drift more and more into depression and inactivity with all the attendant problems.

Then the physician starts experimenting with anti-anxiety drugs and antidepressants. Their patients become addicted. The side effects of the drugs add additional problems. If the fibromyalgia sufferer attempts to discontinue medications, he or she is hit with the added challenge known as "withdrawal symptoms." Patients often move from one doctor or therapist to another—whose treatments vary, but are all unsuccessful. The sufferers often feel trapped inside their bodies, with no freedom in sight.

Who Gets Fibromyalgia?

About 80% of those who suffer from fibromyalgia are women between ages 25 and 55. No one really knows why it affects mostly women. According to Dr. Goldenberg, a professor of medicine and chief of rheumatology at a Boston medical center, about 3 to 6 million Americans are affected. In fact, it is regarded as the most common cause of generalized mus-

4

cle soreness, affecting about 2% of the general population. Men, when afflicted, are not as hard hit as women.

According to available statistics, fibromyalgia affects people between the ages of 20 and 60 years, the incidence peaking at about age 35.

Children and Fibromyalgia

A so-called "juvenile primary fibromyalgia" is reported in about 2% of school children, mostly girls. Symptoms in children include irritability and attention deficit in school. Others complain of allergy problems and painful joints.

Economic Cost of Fibromyalgia

Dr. Wolfe and associates have determined from their studies that it costs the nation about $16 million in missed work and disability payments or poor work performance.

Can Fibromyalgia Be Inherited?

A *CBS Health Watch* article reports that about 28% of offspring of fibromyalgia sufferers (mothers) also developed symptoms. Another study claims 66% of parents of children with fibromyalgia exhibited some consistent muscular pain. But most researchers agree that studies could not conclusively determine whether psychological conditioning by regular contact played a role or whether fibromyalgia is, in fact, generated by genetic factors.

Who Is At Risk?

Although everyone is at risk, it is mostly women between the ages of 25 and 55, especially those with a medical history of trauma. Christine's whiplash injury was her fibromyalgia triggering factor. Other factors might include constant mental aggravation due to frequent relationship discords, and physical, emotional or sexual abuse. Those with low stress tolerance or poor coping capacity are particularly susceptible to fibromyalgia.

How Does Fibromyalgia Progress?

We deduce from several long-term studies that fibromyalgia is chronic in nature, often alternating from "good days" to "bad days." Some sufferers have been forced to stop working altogether.

Although fibromyalgia is chronic, it does not appear to be progressive or fatal. Many people have been known to improve following well-controlled self-help remedies, stress management and fitness programs. Children with fibromyalgia usually improve faster than adults do, probably due to their resilient spirits and active lifestyles.

CHAPTER 2

~

Common Symptoms
and Associated Conditions

There are many diseases that can be confused with fibromyalgia. These have similar symptoms but are technically
not fibromyalgia. This distinction will become more explicit
when we discuss the American College of Rheumatology's diagnostic criteria later in the text.

Similar Conditions That Are Easily Confused
with Fibromyalgia Syndrome Include:

- Chronic fatigue syndrome;
- Lyme disease;
- Lupus;
- Polymyalgia rheumatica;
- Rheumatoid diseases;
- Sjögren's syndrome.

We shall now briefly describe these conditions, their simi-
larities with fibromyalgia and how you can tell them apart.
Please note that fibromyalgia can also come in combination
with one of a whole retinue of diseases. For instance, one may,
in fact, have fibromyalgia syndrome with arthritis or Sjögren's
syndrome, etc. I think this is most often the case. People with
autoimmune problems or connective tissue diseases like
polymyalgia, etc. are particularly prone to fibromyalgia. Often,

physicians fail to check for these other conditions, and, as a result, patients may not improve or respond to medications as they should.

Chronic Fatigue Syndrome

Many of the symptoms of chronic fatigue syndrome (CFS) are quite similar to those of fibromyalgia syndrome (FMS). A major difference is that while fatigue is the dominant symptom in CFS, widespread pain and tender points are more predominant in FMS. Another difference is that cognitive impairment is more pronounced in CFS than in FMS. A similarity, though, is that both FMS and CFS occur in age groups of approximately 20 to 50 years of age, and mostly in women. According to Dr. Carol Jessop, the two syndromes may have similar symptoms, such as:

- Chronic fatigue;
- Memory problems;
- Depressive moods;
- Frequent urination;
- Cold extremities;
- Sleep abnormality;
- Problems with balance;
- Muscle spasm;
- Dry mouth;
- Headaches;
- Muscle aches.

In general, chronic fatigue syndrome is characterized by extreme and continuous fatigue. A little physical exertion usually provokes a fatigue that can incapacitate patients for days. There is no clinical testing for CFS. Instead, physicians endeavor to exclude other conditions before making a diagnosis of chronic fatigue syndrome.

Lyme Disease

Lyme disease is caused by a bacteria called *Borrelia burgdorferi,* usually transmitted by tiny deer ticks. It got its name from the Lyme community in Connecticut, where it was first discovered and named in 1975.

Symptoms begin as a large red spot on the thigh or buttocks, trunk or armpit that expands to about 6 inches in diameter. Other smaller red spots may appear later. Other symptoms include fatigue, chills and fever, muscle and joint pain, headaches or neck stiffness.

Diagnosis of Lyme disease can be difficult as the bacteria is difficult to culture. So diagnosis is usually based on a history of exposure to tick infestation and a measuring of the level of antibodies to Borrelia in the blood of patients.

Lupus

Lupus, which affects about 2 of every 1000 persons, may be diagnosed mistakenly for fibromyalgia. Common symptoms of this disease include joint pains, fatigue, muscle soreness and skin rashes. It has been shown in research studies that about 30% of lupus patients also have fibromyalgia.

Differences from fibromyalgia include: evidence of true joint swelling (arthritis), mouth sores, fever, skin rashes, hair loss, and organ disease like blood in urine. Other characteristics of lupus include elevated blood sedimentation rates, depressed white blood cell count, and increased anti-DNA antibodies.

Fibromyalgia, on the other hand, does not have any of the above findings and is characterized by more widespread pain, tender points and possibly irritable bowel syndrome.

Polymyalgia Rheumatica (PMR)

One difference between fibromyalgia and PMR is that the latter occurs in people over age 50, but, like fibromyalgia, it is more common in women than in men. PMR is a condition that is characterized by severe pain and stiffness in the neck and in the muscles of the shoulders and hips. It can be accompanied by another condition called temporal (giant cell) arteritis. Other symptoms of PMR include fever, weight loss and depression. Onset of symptoms can be either sudden or gradual. A blood test usually reveals a high erythrocyte sedimentation rate.

Rheumatoid Diseases

Rheumatoid arthritis is an autoimmune condition characterized by symmetrical inflammation of joints, usually of the hands and feet, and the eventual disruption of interior joint structures like cartilage, bones and ligaments. A major difference with fibromyalgia is that in fibromyalgia there is neither a joint inflammation nor disruption.

Sjögren's Syndrome

Many patients have been diagnosed with both Sjögren's syndrome and fibromyalgia syndrome. Sjögren's syndrome's cause is unknown. It is characterized by a distinctive type of dry mouth and dry eyes. There are teeth problems, oral infections, difficulty in swallowing. It is an autoimmune problem, prevalent in middle-aged women. Additionally, Sjögren's disease may be associated with arthritis, muscle inflammation, and thyroid and kidney problems. Sometimes patients suffer fatigue and sleep disorders as well.

Diagnostic criteria for Sjögren's disease include evidence of keratoconjunctivitis sica (abnormality and deficiency of tear ducts), autoimmune problems and increased sensitivity to light. Corneal erosion can develop with prolonged dryness of the eyes.

Common Symptoms of Fibromyalgia and Associated Disorders

The following are some common problems fibromyalgia sufferers may have, with their approximate incidence in percentage of patients. Please note that investigators' reports vary percentage-wise and these numbers should be used only as rough estimates.

- Widespread muscle pain or soreness (100%);
- Fatigue (85%);
- Sleep disorders (80%);
- Morning stiffness (75%);

- Headaches (70%);
- Depression and anxiety (20%–50%);
- Irritable bowel syndrome (IBS) and other abdominal and digestive problems (70%);
- Restless legs syndrome (RLS) (31%);
- Cognitive and memory impairment problems (71%);
- Irritable bladder syndrome (12%);
- Pelvic pain (40%);
- Temporomandibular joint dysfunction (TMJ) (25%);
- Vision problems (95%);
- Hearing problems (31%);
- Respiratory problems (33%);
- Hypersensitivity to so-called environmental stressors (50%);
- Raynaud's phenomenon (38%).

Widespread Muscle Pain and Soreness

There may be many other reasons why fibromyalgia sufferers "hurt all over, all the time," but the most common reasons are:

- Lack of refreshing sleep;
- Constant muscle tension.

The problems associated with sleep and the lack of it will be discussed later in greater detail, but in general and under normal circumstances, the normal muscle micro-trauma is repaired naturally during the deep phase of sleep. Absent this phase, fibromyalgia patients' muscle trauma is not repaired, which results in their feeling the soreness about which they so often complain.

Normal muscle tension is the state of readiness of a muscle fiber just before it twitches and performs an action. Because of stress, muscle fibers in the muscles of FMS sufferers are constantly twitching. To put it another way, they are in constant states of readiness, which, in the long term, places them in permanent states of tension. Consequently more blood flow, with its oxygen and nutrients, is required to maintain this habitual tension. Unfortunately, this tension constricts the blood vessels, further diminishing the blood flow that is so badly needed. This results in a lack of oxygen and an accumulation of harmful by-products of muscle activity called *metabolites*, like lactic acid. Metabolites contribute to the sensation of pain in the muscles.

Fatigue

The cause and nature of fatigue in fibromyalgia are complex and multifaceted. The onset of fatigue is easily triggered by slight physical exertion or mental and psychological stress. Scientific evidence indicates fatigue in fibromyalgia is often caused by the following: non-restful sleep; depression and anxiety; lack of physical activity and deconditioning; poor stress management; and hormonal imbalance.

Sleep Disorders

There are 5 phases of sleep in a normal sleep pattern. They are known as stages 1 through 4 and REM (rapid eye movement). The normal sleep cycle progresses from stage 1 through REM stage, then starts all over again from stage 1. Fifty percent of sleep time is spent in stage 2; about 20% in REM stage and the remaining 30% distributed amongst the other three stages. Infants, however, spend most of their time in the REM stage.

Characteristics of the Stages

Stage 1: Sleep is light and one can be awakened easily. Eye movements and muscle activity decrease in speed.

Stage 2: Eye movements stop altogether. Brain activity diminishes to occasional spikes, known as *sleep spindles.*

Stage 3: The brain activity decreases and is measured in a wave form known as delta waves, and interspersed with smaller and faster waves.

Stage 4: Mostly delta wave activity. Difficult to awaken someone in this phase. This is the *deepest sleep* phase, which actually starts toward the latter phase of stage 3.

REM: This stage is characterized by rapid breathing, which is also shallow and irregular; temporary limb and muscle paralysis; rapid eye movements; increased heart rate; and regular dreaming.

The initial REM stage occurs after about 70 to 90 minutes after one falls asleep. The whole sleep cycle is 90 to 110 minutes. The first complete cycle has a relatively short REM stage and a longer deep sleep phase. As sleep progresses, the REM stage increases in duration, while deep sleep stages shorten.

With fibromyalgia patients, there is a sleep disorder called *alpha-EEG anomaly,* in which the patient falls asleep normally, but the deep phase, i.e., stage 4, is often interrupted by awake-like brain activity bursts.

Other sleep disorders include sleep myoclonus (nighttime involuntary jerking of limbs), restless legs syndrome and bruxism (teeth grinding).

Sleep is most restful during the delta or stage 4 phase. This is also called the restorative stage because it is during this stage that "repairing" growth hormones are released from the pituitary gland. This hormone has a direct effect on the regeneration of muscle tissue. FMS patients feel muscle soreness and fatigue in the morning because they have not experienced restorative sleep.

Morning Stiffness

The FMS patient feels each morning as if her muscles are glued down and immobile. This symptom often persists for more than 30 minutes. As explained above, this is a result of a lack of restorative sleep among sufferers.

Headaches

Most FMS sufferers complain of migraine headaches. This is defined as a one-sided and throbbing head pain accompanied by nausea and hypersensitivity to light and sound. The

13

headaches are often triggered by certain kinds of food or strong smells, and may occur during menstruation.

The other commonly experienced type of headache is called a *tension headache*. It is characterized by pain around the head (as if the patient were wearing a hatband) and neck regions. The pain is constant, often precipitated by stress and muscle tension, and usually occurs later in the day.

Recent research studies implicate a high level of substance P, a sensory transmitter that modulates pain perception, as the culprit in headaches of fibromyalgia. This substance has some relevance in the etiology of fibromyalgia and may be why fibromyalgia is usually accompanied by headaches and migraines.

Depression and Anxiety

Most researchers believe fibromyalgia is not a psychiatric disorder. The symptoms of depression are perceived as reactions to or frustration with fibromyalgia and the lifestyle changes it forces on the sufferers.

Irritable Bowel Syndrome (IBS)

The Digestive Diseases Department if the National Institutes of Health (NIH) defines IBS as a disorder of the intestines which leads to cramping pain, bloating, gassiness, and bowel habit changes. Its cause is unknown, and a complete cure is yet to be found.

The colon is about 6 feet long and connects the small intestine with the rectum and anus. Its major function is to absorb water and salts from digestive material that enters from the small intestine. Food may remain for several days in the intestine while most of the salt and fluids are absorbed into the body. The digestive material's residue then passes through the colon by a pattern of colon movements, which further advance the material until it can be evacuated as feces. Colon motility is controlled by nerve and hormonal activity.

Irritable bowel syndrome patients experience is a disorder of the motility of the entire gastrointestinal system. This produces abdominal pain, constipation or diarrhea.

This disorder affects more women than men in a ratio of 3 to 1. It is especially sensitive to stress, diet, certain drugs, hormones and other intestinal irritants.

Normal gut contractions occur at about 6 cycles per minute. In IBS, contractions occur at about 3 cycles per minute. Symptoms include a difficulty in passing stools, leading to painful diarrhea or constipation, or a combination of both.

Some foods, like chocolate and milk, can provoke symptoms. IBS can be more pronounced during menstruation, and perhaps this is why some researchers believe reproductive hormones may be causative factors.

Restless Legs Syndrome (RLS)

This refers to a problem FMS patients may experience, usually in the evening before bedtime. Sufferers experience uncomfortable sensations like numbness, itching, tingling or a crawling sensation in the limbs, sometimes with spontaneous, uncontrollable leg movements.

Cognitive or Memory Impairments (Fibro-fog)

FMS patients often forget things more frequently than is normal. Also decreased is attention span, reflecting a lack of concentration, and a need for more time to process information. The causes of this problem may be attributable to the mental stress and other psychological problems these patients are going through.

Irritable Bladder Syndrome

This syndrome is characterized as an increase in frequency of urination and a chronic feeling of pain and pressure in the lower abdomen. Also experienced are painful urination and some incontinence.

Pelvic Pain

FMS patients often complain about painful menstruation and frequent pain and discomfort in the pelvic area.

Temporomandibular Joint Dysfunction (TMJ)

FMS patients often experience substantial pain in the face and head, occurring in the area of the temporomandibular joint. This is usually caused by spasms of surrounding muscles and ligaments. There may not be an internal joint problem. This condition is also called myofascial pain syndrome. Pain originates in the ear region and spreads to the rest of the face.

Vision and Hearing Problems

Symptoms include sensations of blurring, bouncing or double vision. Hearing problems may comprise hypersensitivity to certain types of sound.

Respiratory Problems

Patients often complain about shortness of breath, even when at rest. Breathing patterns can become erratic and irregular with only minimal exertion.

Hypersensitivity to So-Called Environmental Stressors

The fibromyalgia patient's senses are highly sensitized and susceptible to several environmental stimuli. Cold water or a cold draft from an open window is known to trigger a barrage of symptoms.

Known physical stressors include repetitive activities; abnormal postures; prolonged periods in one posture; or sustained isometric position in daily activities like typing or data entry.

FMS patients are known to have poor stress coping ability. They often break down over little problems. They are often described by family members as "cranky" or "nagging."

Raynaud's Phenomenon

This is also called "cold-induced vasospasm." In lay terms, the small blood vessels constrict, thereby decreasing blood flow to the extremities. The fingers turn very white when exposed to cold temperatures.

CHAPTER 3

~

How Is Fibromyalgia Syndrome Diagnosed?

Diagnosing fibromyalgia syndrome may be compared to peeling off the layers of an onion bulb. Part of the reason why the word "syndrome" is added to it is that it usually comes with several symptoms and associated conditions.

In order to make a correct diagnosis of fibromyalgia, the rheumatologist or physician must exclude other fibromyalgia-like diseases like lupus, chronic fatigue syndrome, rheumatic diseases, Lyme disease, polymyalgia rheumatica, and Sjögren's syndrome, among others described in Chapter 2.

Fibromyalgia is unique in that there is no active inflammation as occurs in rheumatic diseases and tests will usually produce negative results. The physician will usually order a whole range of tests with the intent to exclude other diseases. Some of these tests include extensive blood work, thyroid and liver function tests, antibody detection tests, sedimentation rates and psychological tests.

Past medical, personal and social histories are conducted to determine issues such as past diseases and treatment, physical injuries, episodes of infection, instances of sexual, physical and emotional abuse, nature of current relationships, medical history, etc.

According to the American College of Rheumatology's 1990 criteria, a diagnosis of fibromyalgia syndrome can be made if the following conditions are present:

1. Widespread or generalized muscle pain in more than one extremity that lasts for more than 3 months;

2. A minimum of 11 out of 18 tested tender points. To determine the presence of a tender point, pain must be provoked by a palpation pressure of about 4 km/cm³. Pain must be enough to cause the patient to flinch or pull back. (See Figure 3 for anatomic locations of tender points.)

A trigger point can be differentiated from a tender point because a trigger point pain is dull and usually refers to pain in an area that is distal to the area being palpated. Myofascial pain, for instance, is a localized area of several trigger points.

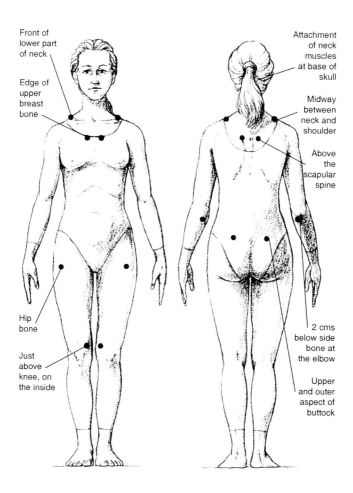

Front of
lower part
of neck

Edge of
upper
breast
bone

Attachment
of neck
muscles
at base of
skull

Midway
between
neck and
shoulder

Above
the
scapular
spine

Hip
bone

Just
above
knee, on
the inside

2 cms
below side
bone at
the elbow

Upper
and outer
aspect of
buttock

Figure 3: Anatomic sites of tender points associated with fibromyalgia syndrome. For a tender point to be confirmed, the patient must wince when a force of about 4 kg/cm³ is applied—or enough pressure sufficient to cause blanching of testing fingernails (not the thumb).

19

CHAPTER 4

~

What Causes
Fibromyalgia Syndrome?

Nobody really knows the specific cause of fibromyalgia. To date, there is no consensus among fibromyalgia researchers as to a single cause for this syndrome. Rather, there are several theories to explain the causes this multi-symptom and multi-faceted heath problem. Some of the more important theories discuss the inclusion of:

* Hereditary factors;
* Chronic sleep disorder;
* Abnormal brain function and neurotransmitter regulation;
* Autoimmune disorder;
* Post-traumatic stress disorder;
* Trauma, like whiplash injury;
* Muscle cell abnormality
* Low levels of Vitamin B_{12};
* High homocysteine levels in the cerebrospinal fluid;
* Viral infection.

Hereditary Factors

A familial predisposition to fibromyalgia has been observed by some investigators. One study reported that 28% of children of mothers with fibromyalgia later developed symptoms of FMS. About 60% developed some kind of fibromyalgia-like muscle pain. Other researchers are not so sure about the veracity of this theory. There is some doubt as to whether it is genetic or simply a psychological sensitization due to close association and sympathy with the patient with fibromyalgia.

Chronic Sleep Disorder

Chronic sleep disturbance may be the precipitating cause of fibromyalgia. As we stated earlier, lack of restorative sleep prevents the action of the pituitary gland responsible for repairing injured muscle tissue. This leads to muscle hypoxia (oxygen deficiency), and accumulation of metabolites like lactic acid. This problem consequently leads to constant feelings of muscle soreness and pain.

Abnormal Brain Function
and Neurotransmitter Regulation

This condition is characterized by the following:

- Brain tissue studies and scans have revealed limited blood flow to pain regulation areas of the brain.

- There may be possible abnormalities with the internal brain system that controls functions like sleep, growth, stress response and depressive moods. These organs include pituitary, adrenal glands and hypothalamus.

- Very high levels of somatomedin C responsible for informing the brain about pain-producing stimuli. High levels of somatomedin C produce increased sensitivity to noxious stimuli in fibromyalgia patients.

- Low levels of the neurotransmitter serotonin and its building material called *tryptophan*. Neurotransmitters act as chemical messengers between brain neurons. Low levels of these chemical messengers are known to be associated with depressive moods, headaches and migraines, and gastrointestinal problems.

- Elevated levels of substance P in the cerebrospinal fluid have been implicated in fibromyalgia. Animal studies indicate that high levels of substance P lead to what is called "central sensitization." Substance P is known to decrease the threshold of synaptic sensitivity so that the central nervous system reaction to minor stimuli becomes exaggerated. This is why fibromyalgia patients experience pain very easily.

Autoimmune Disorder

This condition is brought about by a defective immune system that produces agents known as *autoantibodies.* These autoantibodies attack the body's own proteins, mistaking them for harmful foreign proteins. Several of these autoantibodies have been discovered in FMS patients.

Post-traumatic Stress Disorder

Medical and social histories of many fibromyalgia sufferers indicate incidents of past sexual, physical or emotional abuse. These incidents create varied anxiety disorders that lead to a full-blown condition known as post-traumatic stress disorder (PTSD). This condition is characterized by several fibromyalgia symptoms, including sleeplessness, mood problems, cognitive problems and muscle pain.

Trauma

Fibromyalgia is often precipitated by trauma. A report appearing in the *Fibromyalgia Wellness Letter,* a publication of the Arthritis Foundation, indicates that some scientists in Israel were able to connect the incidence of neck injuries with fibromyalgia. In general, most fibromyalgia patients report a history of past trauma. How trauma provokes fibromyalgia syndrome is not yet fully understood.

Muscle Cell Abnormality

One theory proposed that FMS patients have lower levels of ATP (adenosine triphosphate) and phosphocreatine in their muscle cells. These enzymes are responsible for the in-and-out movement of calcium through muscle cells than other people do. Calcium motion is a very important process in normal muscle contraction. With lowered ATP levels, calcium ions are not moved back into the cell after muscle contraction. As a result these fibers remain "frozen" in contraction. They fail to "relax." Some researchers believe the problem may not be within the muscle, but may be a problem within the hormonal and nervous system.

Low Levels of Vitamin B$_{12}$ and High Levels of Homocysteine in Cerebrospinal Fluid

The *Scandinavian Journal of Rheumatology* reported on a study of 12 female patients with both fibromyalgia and chronic fatigue syndrome. Dr. Regland and associates compared this group to the control group of 18 healthy women. They found that the fibromyalgia and chronic fatigue subjects' cerebrospinal fluid contained a significant amount of homocysteine and a lower amount of Vitamin B$_{12}$ than that of the normal subjects. High levels of homocysteine have been implicated in cardiovascular problems and other diseases as well. Homocysteine is degraded in enzyme reactions called transsulfuration and remethylation to form methionine, which is the building block for SAM-e formation. Vitamin B$_{12}$ is very important in these enzymatic processes.

Viral Infection

There is a theory that fibromyalgia may be caused by a viral infection. According to Dr. Leon Chaitow, a practitioner and senior lecturer at the Center for Community Care and Primary Health, University of Westminster, London, UK, latent viruses may be reactivated by release of chemicals known as cytokines. This triggers off the "flu-like" symptoms often associated with fibromyalgia. Researchers are yet to discover the elusive virus involved in fibromyalgia.

CHAPTER 5

~

Conventional Pharmacologic Treatment of Fibromyalgia

To date, no single medication has been approved by the FDA for the treatment of fibromyalgia symptoms. Because of this, doctors use the same medications used to treat rheumatic diseases that share some symptoms with fibromyalgia. But unlike rheumatic diseases, fibromyalgia does not have an active inflammatory process. This leads to some difficulty for the physician and risks for the patient, since appropriate dosage guidelines and side effect information are not available to the physician. According to Dr. Jon Russell, medications are chosen and prescribed based mainly on a pragmatic basis and no particular medication is regarded as a cure.

Some of the Most Common Complaints and Their Most Commonly Prescribed Treatments

Sleep Disorders

Common medications used include

- Tricyclics (Elavil, Sinequan, Trazodone, etc.)
- Sedatives and anxiolytics (Xanax, Ambien, etc.)
- Klonopin (prescribed for restless legs syndrome or myoclonus)

Fatigue

- SSRIs (selective serotonin reuptake inhibitors) like Prozac, Zoloft, Paxil, etc. are often prescribed for fatigue and depressive moods

Irritable Bowel Syndrome (IBS)

- Bentyl
- Levsin (used to relieve pain from intestinal spasms, cramps and diarrhea)
- dietary fiber
- Urised (used as a mild anesthetic that affects the nerves that control the action of smooth muscles)

Headaches

- For recurring tension-type headaches, doctors often prescribe a mixture of muscle relaxants and painkillers, or a combination of analgesic-barbiturate and caffeine.
- For persistent migraine, the following are often used: zolmitriptan (Zomig), sumatriptan (Imitrex) and rizatriptan (Maxalt).
- NSAIDs (non-steroidal anti-inflammatory drugs) like Relafen, naproxen, ibuprofen, etc.

According to Dr. Russell, fibromyalgia patients are usually given a combination of NSAIDs and an anxiolytic or a low dose of a tricyclic antidepressant like amitriptyline or cyclobenzaprine.

To avoid the stomach problems caused by NSAIDs, another similar-acting drug called celecoxib (Celebrex) can be used. Celebrex is new in the market, and is being hailed as a "super aspirin." It is as effective as ibuprofen and other NSAIDs.

Modes of Action of Common Drugs Used to Treat Fibromyalgia

Tricyclic Antidepressants

As the name suggests, tricyclics have a 3-ring chemical structure. They were first introduced into the American market in 1960, for relief of depressive moods. Tricyclics work by preventing the reuptake of the neurotransmitters serotonin and norepinephrine, while activating them.

Tricyclics usually require 10 to 14 days on a regular dose to start working. Full effect may be delayed for up to 6 weeks.

Common tricyclic antidepressants:

- Amitriptyline (Elavil);
- Imipramine (Imavate, Presamine, Tofranil);
- Doxepin (Adapin, Sinequan);
- Desipramine (Norpramin, Pertofrane);
- Protriptyline (Surmontil);
- Anafranil (Clomipramine).

SSRIs (Selective Serotonin Reuptake Inhibitors)

This group of antidepressants has effects similar to tricyclics, except they act to prevent the reuptake of only serotonin. Introduced on the American market in 1998, they are the most recent group of medications used to treat fatigue in fibromyalgia.

Common SSRIs are:

- Fluoxetine (Prozac);
- Sertraline (Zoloft);
- Paroxetine (Paxil).

NSAIDs (Non-Steroidal Anti-Inflammatory Drugs)

NSAIDs have a dual function. First, they affect the prostaglandin system, which is involved in the sensation of pain. Second, they act to reduce inflammation. They are frequently used to reduce fibromyalgia headaches.

Common examples include:

- Relafen;
- Naproxen;
- Ibuprofen.

Anxiolytics—Also called Sedatives and Tranquilizers
Mostly prescribed to relieve and manage anxiety disorders, they act by relaxing muscles and reducing tension. Used in fibromyalgia to relieve sleeplessness. A common example includes a group called benzodiazepines. Examples of long-acting ones include:

- Diazepam (Valium);
- Alprazolam (Xanax);
- Chlordiazepoxide (Librium).

Short-acting benzodiazepines include:

- Lorazapam (Ativan);
- Temazepam (Restoril);
- Oxazepam (Serax).

PART 2

Re-evaluating
Your Medications

CHAPTER 6

~

Your Medications May Be Doing You More Harm Than Good

According to a recent article in the *American Journal of Hospital Pharmacy,* the major reasons medications are prescribed include:

- To enhance the patient's current quality of life by reducing disease symptoms;
- To arrest and regress the disease;
- To prevent disease/symptoms from occurring or recurring.

But your medication can become a double-edged sword. It can remove symptoms, and perhaps temporarily mask them, or it can become a foreign agent in the body, having displaced natural ones from their receptor sites, and could even form a *totally new adverse compound,* further complicating your current problems.

Various medical studies recently have highlighted the issue, which they call "the silent epidemic." According to J. Lazarou and associates' 1998 study, reported in the *Journal of the American Medical Association,* medications are known to cause serious adverse effects that can cause disabilities or even fatalities. According to the report, 106,000 fatalities occur from drug adverse effects yearly. As a cause of death, it could rank as the fifth highest in the nation. Furthermore, medication-related adverse reactions cost the nation about $85 billion annually.

There is ample scientific evidence that the use of large doses of psychoactive medications for long periods of time for a chronic, vaguely-known condition like fibromyalgia is not good medical practice, especially when alternative patient-empowering remedies can be prescribed. According to Dr. Breggin, modern medicine does not yet have a handle on the manner in which the human brain functions. We are yet to understand the nature of its myriad internal interconnections, the numerous types of chemical messengers known as neuro-transmitters. Most importantly, we don't fully understand how a foreign chemical, like an antidepressant, can act on so delicate and sensitive a structure as the human brain. According to Dr. Breggin, our knowledge of these issues "is largely limited to test-tube studies of biochemical reactions utilizing ground-up pieces of animal brain. We simply do not understand the overall impact of drugs on the brain." Some of the so-called studies on which we base our decision to prescribe may very well be marketing propaganda orchestrated by the profit-crazy and exceedingly influential drug manufacturing companies, who have much at stake in our continued and mass usage of such drugs.

According to Drs. Gillian Buttler and Tony Hope, in their book *Managing Your Mind,* long-term use of tranquilizers can create the following problems:

1. *It can prevent you from finding long-lasting solutions to your problems.* In the short run, they can help you relax, sleep better for the night, and cope for a couple of days until the pressure builds up again. However, it does not address the underlying sources of your stress and problems. The medication may offer merely a temporary utopia from the real problems of life that need to be dealt with, such as poor relationship issues, high levels of stress and muscle/tension coping problems.

2. *You end up with a psychological dependence on your medications.* You can't leave home without them. If you realize you have done so, you go into a panic, afraid you won't be able to cope without them.

3. *You can get addicted physiologically to your medications.* It is usually easier to start than to quit. If you ever try to quit after a long-term usage, you will be hit with a barrage of withdrawal symptoms. Your life is no longer under your control and you get caught up in a vicious cycle of which you feel you have no hope of escaping.

4. *Long-term antidepressant usage dulls your feelings.* People soon notice you are no longer your old self. That natural zest for life and the spontaneous reactions to the vicissitudes of life soon become things of the past.

Too many physicians make decisions too quickly to prescribe psychoactive drugs. They spend about 15 minutes making a decision that changes their patient's life forever. There have been reported instances in which physicians changed their prescribing stance or philosophy totally after becoming patients themselves and trying these drugs. How would anybody really know, if they had not tried them out themselves?

The problem, I tend to believe, is aided by the patient's eagerness for a "quick fix" to her problems, as many people are intolerant of the slightest discomfort or pain. And it wouldn't make good business sense for the private practice physician to resist the patient's craving for tranquilizers. According to Gabriele Rico, in *Pain and Possibility: Writing Your Way Through Personal Crisis,* "The awareness that pain and possibility are interdependent . . . seeing them as extremes of a single continuum instead of opposites, we begin to see the potential for growth inherent in pain."

Perhaps your pain may be an opportunity for a serious lifestyle conversion in all of its spiritual, emotional and physical ramifications.

CHAPTER 7

~

Adverse Effects and Withdrawal Symptoms Associated with Drugs Used to Treat Fibromyalgia Syndrome

Adverse Effects of Antidepressants

The adverse side effects of all antidepressants can be grouped under the following headings:

- Anticholinergic effects;
- Cardiovascular effects;
- Renal effects;
- Sexual problems;
- Otolaryngeal problems;
- Skin and allergic reactions;
- Central nervous system effects.

Following is a clarification of each of these potential side effects.

Anticholinergic Effects

- Memory impairments and sometimes confusion;
- Lowered blood pressure;
- Episodes of dry mouth;
- Bowel problems leading to constipation;
- Urination difficulties, like pain or delayed urination;
- Blurring of vision and drying of eyes.

Cardiovascular Effects

- Low blood pressure resulting in dizziness;
- Heart palpitations;
- Death can result from cardiac arrhythmias.

Gastrointestinal Effects

- Altered bowel movements leading to constipation;
- Nausea and vomiting;
- Diarrhea;
- Patient may gain weight due to increase in appetite and food intake (tricyclics) or lose weight (SSRIs).

Renal Effects

This would include urinary retention and difficulty.

Sexual Effects

- Decreased libido;
- Impotence and diminished sexual arousal;
- Swelling of the testicles;
- Possible enlargement of breasts in both sexes.

Otolaryngeal Problems

- Nasal congestion;
- Drying of eyes and vision problems;
- Glaucoma.

Skin and Allergic Reactions

- There may be increased or decreased swelling;
- Allergic reactions may occur with skin rashes.

Central Nervous System Effects

- Drowsiness;

- Impaired ability to concentrate or remember things;

- Muscle tremors, slurring of speech, seizures, nightmares and restlessness.

Many research studies seem to agree that even though anti-depressants may offer short-term benefits for fibromyalgia sufferers, in the long term, they create other serious problems. Even the good short-term benefits wear off within a few months. Some patients, like Jean (reported in the *Fibromyalgia Wellness Letter*), who has had fibromyalgia for more than 10 years, experienced flashbacks, depressive moods and panic attacks with even a low dose of tricyclics, and weight gain. Fibromyalgia sufferers seem to experience fewer side effects with the SSRIs (Prozac, Zoloft) than with the tricyclics (Elavil, Endep, Sinequan, etc.).

In his book *Talking Back to Prozac: What Doctors Aren't Telling You About Today's Most Controversial Drug,* Dr. Breggin stated that Prozac can have extreme side effects like *akathisia,* restless legs syndrome and the continual need to pace. Scientific studies confirm this problem in about 10% to 25% of all those on Zoloft. The restless legs problem may be something fibromyalgia patients should discuss with their doctors if they are on Prozac. Prozac, in extreme cases, has been linked to suicidal acts and aggressive behaviors towards other people.

Adverse Effects of NSAIDs
(Non-Steroidal Anti-Inflammatory Drugs)

Chances for adverse effects increase when two or more NSAIDs are taken together over a long period of time, or if you take them with alcoholic beverages.

These drugs can cause confusion, dizziness and light-headedness in some people. Others may become extra sensitive to sunlight, resulting in sunburns with slight exposure.

RE-EVALUATING YOUR MEDICATIONS

Serious side effects include gastrointestinal problems—upset stomach, ulcers, stomach cramps, nausea, heartburn or vomiting of blood.

Adverse Effects of Anxiolytics or Tranquilizers Like Benzodiazepines (Oxazepam, Alprazolam, etc.)

These include:

- Low blood pressure, dizziness and light-headedness;
- Bronchospasm;
- Raynaud's phenomenon—cold fingers and toes;
- Dry mouth and nasal congestion;
- Urination problems;
- Central nervous system effects resulting in disorientation and confusion; memory problems; frequent episodes of uncontrollable anger.

Common Withdrawal Reactions of Antidepressants and Anxiolytics Used to Treat Fibromyalgia Patients

One of the most important reasons *not* to get on any addictive medication is the withdrawal reaction. You will definitely have withdrawal if you decide to stop. It's like someone deciding to climb a treacherous mountain, who should also consider how she will come down. There will be no helicopters to carry her off the summit. It is something only she can do. Also be aware that some physicians are not fully informed about withdrawal reactions, coming from a treatment philosophy background of regular prescription and maintenance. According to Mosher and Biroti, in their book *Community Mental Health: Principles and Practice,* "a sizeable minority of physicians denied being confidently aware of the existence of antidepressant withdrawal symptoms." In the final analysis, it is your body, your mind and your life. You must take charge of them.

All antidepressants and anti-anxiety medications are addictive. Your physician may mistakenly interpret your withdrawal symptoms, should you try to discontinue the medication He may say that "you really need this medication and you have to be on it for the rest of your life." This is not always true. And many conscientious psychiatrists will agree with me.

But the withdrawal reactions can be quite significant, depending on the type of medication, dosage and length of time used. The higher the dosage and the longer the time of usage, the more severe the withdrawal reactions will be. These reactions range from emotional to physical, and can be felt within days of stopping the medication. The short-acting tranquilizers like Ambien, Halcyon or Xanax will cause withdrawal reactions quickly, even in between doses. Withdrawal reactions usually have effects opposite those produced by taking that particular drug. Some of these effects, especially the emotional ones, may last a very long time after completely stopping the medication. It is possible to stop your addictive medication. You just have to want to stop, and find a psychiatrist who will help you stop by a systematic drug withdrawal program.

Benzodiazepine Withdrawal Reactions (Oxazepam, Xanax, etc.)

These can produce the potential for withdrawal reactions even if you discontinue taking them after only a few weeks. Discontinuing Xanax, for example, can cause increased anxiety and panic after only about 8 weeks of use. In general, depending on dosage and length of time used, benzodiazepines will cause the following withdrawal reactions:

- Flu-like symptoms, chills, shivering;
- Stomach upsets like nausea, vomiting and diarrhea;
- Sweating;

- Fatigue and muscle soreness;
- Dizziness;
- Blurred vision;
- Weight loss;
- Psychosis;
- Seizures.

These reactions may appear in any combination and any degree of severity.

Tricyclic Antidepressants Withdrawal Reactions

According to Dr. R.M. Wolfe in his 1997 research study, an attempt to come off tricyclic antidepressants usually triggers a barrage of "bewildering symptoms." Some of these include:

- Emotional problems like depressive moods, manic episodes, reckless and dangerous behaviors, incidents of very poor judgment, etc.;
- Flu-like symptoms;
- Gastrointestinal problems like stomach cramps, vomiting and diarrhea, nausea, loss of appetite, etc.;
- Memory and other cognitive problems like disorientation;
- Uncontrollable muscle movements, such as spasms and restless legs syndrome;
- Sleep problems, including insomnia and vivid dreams;
- Cardiac arrhythmias that can lead to death if sufficiently severe.

SSRI Withdrawal Reactions (Zoloft, Prozac, Celexa or Paxil)

Their withdrawal reactions are similar to those of tricyclics with the following additional problems:

- Balance disorders;
- Sensory disorders;
- Aggressive and impulsive behaviors.

Drs. Breggin and Cohen, in their definitive book on the subject, gave the following case studies:

- A 32-year-old man discontinued Prozac after 6 months of usage and ended up with withdrawal reactions that included painful extensor muscle spasms and uncontrollable tongue-protruding movements.

- A 34-year-old woman tried to stop taking Luvox after she became pregnant. Her withdrawal symptoms included feelings of aggression, like wanting to kill someone.

- Another woman started having problems after reducing her dosage of Zoloft from 100 mg to 50 mg per day. A few days later, she started having profound fatigue and depressive moods, and even entertained suicidal thoughts.

PART 3

∽

SAM-e
to the Rescue

CHAPTER 8

~

What Is SAM-e?

SAM-e (pronounced *sammy*) is not another new drug product, and it's not an herb or hormone. It is a naturally occurring substance, evenly distributed in human tissues. SAM-e has been in the news lately because it is a harmless supplement that scientists have determined to be very beneficial in the treatment of several health conditions, including fibromyalgia. The wonder of SAM-e is that it works faster and even better than regular drugs without producing any side effects, as drugs do.

Its full biochemical name is "S-adenosyl-L-methionine." Quite a mouthful! To make the pronunciation a little easier, scientists abbreviated it to "SAM-e" or "SAM." Its biochemical uniqueness is identified by its chemical structure, which is very versatile and allows it to participate in our bodies' several beneficial metabolic processes.

History of SAM-e

SAM-e was discovered and described by Dr. G. L. Cantoni in 1953, at the National Institutes of Health in Bethesda, Maryland. It is formed by the action of ATP (adenosyn triphosphate) and L-methionine or just "methionine," through the enzymatic action of methionine-adenosyl-transferase. Methionine, the building block of SAM-e, is an essential amino acid that is usually supplemented by a well-balanced and regular diet of soybeans, seeds and lentils, eggs, and protein-rich foods such as fish and meat, a necessary condition for maintaining other supplements such as the B vitamins—B_{12}, B_6, folic acid and a nutrient called TMG (trimethyl-glycine).

Children have about seven times more SAM-e in their blood than adults. Men have a higher level than women. The level of SAM-e is known to decrease with the aging process and has been implicated as a causative factor in disease conditions such as depression, Alzheimer's and Parkinson's diseases.

As I mentioned earlier, the versatile chemical structure of SAM-e enables it to participate in several of the body's metabolic processes. After ATP, SAM-e is the most dynamic single substance in the body. The author of *Methyl Magic,* Dr. Craig Cooney, goes as far as to claim that without SAM-e and the process of methylation, which it mediates, there would be no life as we know it.

Technically, methylation is a metabolic process in which SAM-e donates its methyl group—a very reactive by-product that is enzymatically transferred to a methyl group acceptor. After donating its methyl group, SAM-e becomes a by-product called S-adenosyl homocysteine or SAH. SAH is further degraded by a transfer of its sulfur substrate to other molecules to form several sulfur-containing compounds like cysteine. Cysteine is the building block for another important substance— an antioxidant called glutathione, which I shall discuss later.

Although SAM-e was discovered in 1953, it took a while before a stable form of SAM-e that can exist outside the body could be produced. But in 1973, Dr. Fiechi found a way to do it. He discovered a chemical process that can stabilize SAM-e enough so it can be used in clinical trials. Then, in 1975, Dr. Stramentinoli published the first scientific paper about SAM-e's many pharmacological merits. Finally, in 1976 and 1977, manufacturers obtained patents to produce the stabilized salt forms of SAM-e in the United States.

Part of the reason SAM-e is only recently known in U.S. markets is that most of the scientific investigations and clinical trials were conducted in Europe, notably Italy. Unlike the United

States, Italy is a country that has always been open to alternative forms of healthcare. Nutritionals and supplements have always been parts of the mainstream health care delivery system.

An important milestone in the life history of SAM-e in the United States is the passage of important Congressional legislation in 1994 called the Dietary Supplement Health and Education Act (DSHEA). This new Act allows drug manufacturers to produce and market any supplement with a good safety record without FDA prior authorization, as long as these companies do not make any outrageous claims about the efficacy of these supplements. Among these newly marketable supplements is SAM-e.

There is a drawback to DSHEA, however. There is no longer any quality check scrutiny by the FDA. This permits the dishonest producers to flood the markets with substandard products. The two forms of pharmaceutical grade SAM-e currently available are the *tosylate* (the type commonly imported by U.S. companies) and the *butanedisulfonate* forms. Because SAM-e is absorbed mainly through the intestine, it is usually manufactured in an "enteric coated" tablet form. This allows it to pass intact through the stomach's digestive environment.

SAM-e is very unstable, which means it can easily be broken down by moisture and heat. You must make sure you are buying a well-packaged product that you will store properly, usually in a "cool and dry" environment.

CHAPTER 9

~

How Does
SAM-e Work?

Impact of Methylation on Human Life

Now that we know what SAM-e is and what it is not, the next question is: How does it work its purported magic? The answer lies in the metabolic process well-known among the scientific community called *methylation*. According to a well-known methylation scientist, Dr. Craig Cooney, without methylation, life as we know it would not exist. Another researcher puts it this way: "SAM-e is the single most dynamic substance in the body besides ATP."

Methylation is the metabolic process in which SAM-e donates one or more of its methyl groups (a methyl group consists of one carbon atom joined to three hydrogen atoms) to several "acceptor" molecules, thereby producing several beneficial body compounds. One of the most profound impacts of methylation is in the expression or re-activation of DNA, without which, of course, we would not exist.

DNA (deoxyribonucleic acid) is the policeman of our bodies' zillion cells. It makes sure each is doing what it is supposed to do. One important function it performs is making sure that genes that can produce cancerous states are kept under lock and key. This is the basic reason I consider SAM-e such a very important player in the relief of fibromyalgia syndrome—a condition that most scientists believe is caused and maintained by a central nervous system that has gone berserk.

According to Dr. Cooney, SAM-e, through methylation, is involved in the following beneficial metabolic processes (among others):

- Mediates in the formation of the body's "biological clock" regulator known as melatonin;

- Assists in the manufacture of adrenaline of the "fight or flight" response fame. When we are faced with danger, adrenaline automatically prepares our bodies for action. The heart beats faster, pumping more blood and oxygen into muscle tissues for their usage in fighting or fleeing from danger.

- Assists in the manufacture of several neurotransmitters, such as the transformation of L-dopa into dopamine, which is a principal mood regulator;

- With SAM-e, through transmethylation (a term used interchangeably with methylation), creates many other substances, like L-carnitine, responsible for the transportation of long-chain fatty acids to muscles, where they are utilized as fuel;

- Through the process of methylation, produces *creatine phosphate*. Athletes take supplement forms of creatine phosphate for quick bursts of energy during high-impact sports.

- Through methylation, removes histamine from our systems. Histamine, as we know, is responsible for causing or promoting several allergies and inflammatory reactions.

Scientists believe that the full impact of transmethylation is not yet fully understood. Animal studies indicate that the transport of specific nutrients in both bacteria and the body cells' membrane vesicles is controlled by the level of methylation.

But the story does not end with methylation. After losing its methyl groups, the residue is a compound called S-adenosyl-L-homocysteine (SAH). In a process known as *transsulfuration*, this compound later loses its sulfur substrate to another molecule (with Vitamin B_6 as a co-factor) to form L-cysteine and several other sulfur-containing compounds.

Eventually L-cysteine, through other enzymatic processes, forms the body's major free-radical scavenger, *glutathione.*

Glutathione

As you can see, this powerful antioxidant cannot be produced in our bodies without SAM-e's help. In the absence of antioxidants, free radicals will take control and toxins will overwhelm our bodies. A free radical is an excited "bad guy" roaming the body. This molecule is highly charged. It has an odd number of electrons. An odd number forces the free radical to pair up with and change, or mutate, any kind of atom. Free radicals come from harmful products like food preservatives. These free radicals destroy the body through a process known as oxidation. An antioxidant, therefore, is a substance which "obstructs, restrains or neutralizes" an oxidative element.

Glutathione, together with SAM-e, has its highest concentration in the liver. In the liver, glutathione does more detoxifying than anywhere else in the body. The liver is responsible for the elimination of harmful toxins. Low levels of glutathione could lead to liver toxin overload and eventual failure. SAM-e, therefore, is known to have had beneficial effects in the treatment of liver diseases, since it helps produce glutathione.

Homocysteine: the SAM-e Adversary

High levels of homocysteine can lead to another condition called homocystinuria. High homocysteine levels in the blood have also been known to cause heart disease. SAM-e and homocysteine act on the opposite ends of a precarious balance. A high level of homocysteine is a certain indication of low blood SAM-e levels. Likewise, SAM-e acts promptly to regulate homocysteine levels.

Are There Other Substances that Can Promote the Methylation Process?

Yes. Trimethyl-glycine is another methyl group donor. Its limitation, though, is that it is not known to be involved with methylation within brain cells.

As I mentioned before, the methylation process decreases in tandem with the aging process. Low levels of SAM-e in the blood invariably lead to higher levels of homocysteine and oxidation. So as we age and SAM-e levels in the blood deplete, we will need to supplement with SAM-e.

CHAPTER 10

~

How Does SAM-e Relieve Fibromyalgia Symptoms?

Before discussing the several scientific studies that conclusively offer proofs of the beneficial and symptom-relieving effects of SAM-e on fibromyalgia, I would like to outline some basic facts.

Fibromyalgia is not a simple condition; rather, it is called a syndrome because there are several other problems associated with it. One symptom is common in all sufferers: a kind of augmentation of pain and symptoms. This tends to suggest a problem with the basic descriptors of Life itself—DNA, RNA, polyamines and protein synthesis problems.

As mentioned in earlier chapters, SAM-e, because of its great ability to donate a very reactive methyl group, has become the most versatile and dynamic substance in the body aside from ATP. Without methylation and transsulfuration, of which SAM-e is the main progenitor, Life would not exist.

So, if you are looking for a multifaceted curative agent, SAM-e is your answer. It repairs and it replenishes. Figure 10 outlines the scientific rationale behind SAM-e's probable action in relieving fibromyalgia syndrome symptoms.

SAM-e: A Theoretical Model (see Figure 10)

A. Probable FMS causative factors in which SAM-e may be able to mediate:

- Gene expression abnormality;
- Sleep disorder;

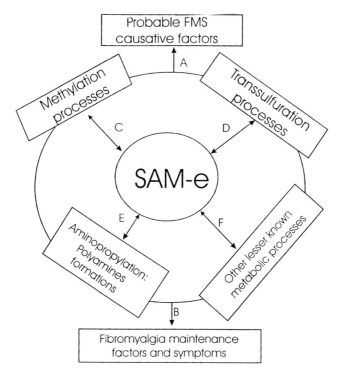

Figure 10: A theoretical model for the probable action of SAM-e in the relief of fibromyalgia symptoms.

- Abnormal brain function and neurotransmitter regulation;
- High homocysteine levels in CSF;
- Autoimmune disorder.

B. Factors and symptoms of fibromyalgia for which SAM-e brings relief:

- Depressive moods and fatigue;
- Muscle pain and tender points;
- Migraine headaches;
- CNS sensory perception abnormalities;
- Histamine and allergens;
- Sleep or circadian rhythm disorders;
- Too many oxidants and toxins in the body.

C. Methylation processes

- Manufacture of neurotransmitters like dopamine, serotonin and melatonin;
- DNA;
- RNA;
- Protein synthesis;
- Phospholipid synthesis and regulation.

D. Transsulfuration processes

- Glutathione formation and antioxidation;
- Cysteine synthesis;
- Taurin.

E. Aminopropylation (Polyamines formations)

Action of SAM-e with arginine to catalyze the synthesis of

- Spermine;

- Spermidine;
- Putrescine.

F. Several other lesser known metabolic processes in which SAM-e acts as a precursor:

- Propylamine component donation after decarboxylation;
- Allosteric factor in several conditions;
- Bacterial DNA restriction and modification;
- *E. coli* restriction and modification;
- Involvement in the reduction of heavy metals—like cobalt or iron—in the process of transforming protein into a catalytically charged enzyme;
- Involved in the modulation of the different actions of norepinephrine and morphine through transmethylation.

The healthcare implications of the above processes in which SAM-e is involved are enormous. In fact, a complete discussion is far beyond the intended scope of this book. However, a more thorough discussion of some topics follows:

Where and How SAM-e Can Help

SAM-E and Gene Expression Abnormality

DNA (deoxyribonucleic acid) is the genetic blueprint of all living organisms. It is found in loosely coiled threads or helixes, called *chromatin*, that congregate to form chromosomes. RNA, mRNA and tRNA (ribonucleic acid, messenger RNA and transfer RNA) are responsible for the sequencing of amino acids in the formation of different protein compounds.

SAM-e, through its methylation of DNA and RNA, activates or deactivates genes, a process which results in their growth and repair. This process has some implications on SAM-e's part in cartilage formation and repair in osteoarthritis.

Activated genes also produce disease-fighting antibodies or regress tumors by gene deactivation. Therefore, an increase in

SAM-e levels in the system of fibromyalgia victims would promote faulty gene repair, cell health and action.

Also, SAM-e plays an important role in the manufacture of polyamines. These molecules contain nitrogen and are intimately involved with DNA and gene expression repairs.

SAM-E and Sleep Disorders

Through methylation, SAM-e reacts with serotonin to manufacture *melatonin*. Secreted by the pineal gland, melatonin is responsible for synchronizing hormonal release. In this way, it regulates the so-called "circadian rhythm." Daylight acts as an enhancer for the release of melatonin, and darkness suppresses its release. Significant scientific evidence shows that an imbalance in the melatonin production would result in insomnia and other sleep disorders.

A theory about aging, according to Dr. Julian Whitaker, is that the body is genetically programmed to wind down like a clock. Thus the balance between daytime and nighttime patterns gets blurred with age. Supplementing with melatonin, according to the doctor, would put "the tick and tock back into your tick-tocks." But you won't need to if you have optimal methylation.

Optimal methylation would also have far-reaching effects on muscle soreness and fatigue experienced by fibromyalgia sufferers resulting from lack of restorative sleep. You see, our bodies are wired up like an electrical circuit. If you disconnect it in one spot, the whole system shuts down.

Another research study worthy of mention is the one conducted in Germany by Offenbacher and associates titled "Possible association of fibromyalgia with a polymorphism in the serotonin transporter gene regulatory region." The method used was to analyze the genomic DNA of 62 patients who have FMS, per the American College of Rheumatology's diagnostic criteria. They also analyzed 110 healthy patients to act as controls. The study found a gene abnormality in fibromyalgia patients that resulted in altered serotonin metabolism. (Serotonin is the precursor of melatonin.)

SAM-E, Abnormal Brain Function and Neurotransmitter Regulation

Several studies claim that toxic substances and metabolites associated with psychiatric disorders arise from a faulty transmethylation process of brain compounds, also known as neurotransmitters. But further studies have narrowed the problem down to a failure in the transmethylation process. This, of course, would have implications for the role of SAM-e in neurotransmitter methylation.

Neurotransmitters that are known to benefit from SAM-e's activity include serotonin, epinephrine, norepinephrine and dopamine. The brain and the whole central nervous system would benefit from SAM-e's phospholipid production, like phosphatidylserine. So proper supplementation with SAM-e by fibromyalgia sufferers and the aged will definitely boost brain phospholipid production.

SAM-E and High CSF Homocysteine Levels

Homocysteine retains a seesaw relationship with SAM-e. A very high level of homocysteine in the cerebrospinal fluid is a certain indication of low levels of SAM-e in the body. Homocysteine, a sulfur-containing compound, can be beneficial in small amounts. Large amounts, however, lead to several diseases that include heart disease, cancer, depression and fibromyalgia. A Swedish study discovered a consistent connection between high levels of homocysteine and low levels of Vitamin B_{12} in cerebrospinal fluid (CSF) of fibromyalgia sufferers.

SAM-E and Autoimmune Disorder

Faulty immune system activation results in excessive productions of immunoglobulins. According to David E. Berg and associates at the ITEMEX Laboratories in Phoenix, Arizona, every chronic fatigue syndrome and fibromyalgia patient they had ever worked with could trace onset to some previous disease state. According to their research, presented at the 1998 American Association of Chronic Fatigue Syndrome Conference, in Cambridge, Massachusetts, the immunoglobulins poke holes through protective protein sheaths inside blood vessels. Consequently, excess thrombin converts fibrinogen into a soluble fibrinogen monomer called fibrin. The coating of the interior lining of these blood vessels blocks normal blood flow of essential oxygen and nutrients, thereby preventing surrounding body tissues from getting them.

SAM-e, through DNA and RNA methylation, has repairing effects on this and other autoimmune problems.

SAM-e and Depressive Moods and Fatigue

There is still some controversy about whether fibromyalgia is caused by depression or other psychiatric states, or whether the fibromyalgia syndrome actually brings about depression. Most likely, sufferers become depressed by the constant pain and low quality of life. Both mental and physical fatigue result from poor, unrestorative sleep. Other known causes of depression include:

- Serotonin deficiency;
- Hormonal system imbalance;
- Thyroid gland underactivity;
- Deficiency of amino acids;
- Nutritional deficiency;
- Weakened immune system;
- Environmental allergies and food sensitivities;
- Poor stress-coping ability;
- Too many toxins and oxidants in the body;
- Inactivity and general deconditioning;
- Inadequate light;

- Stressful relationships;
- Low blood sugar or hypoglycemia;
- Lifestyle issues.

Already, SAM-e has been shown to regulate the action of many of the above-mentioned causative factors of depression. An overwhelming amount of scientific evidence indicates that SAM-e, indeed, would relieve depression even faster and better than regular antidepressants, without leaving behind the usual side effects.

According to the well-known expert in this matter, Dr. Richard Brown, SAM-e is a powerful antidepressant which works gently in the body without the side effects of regular prescription drugs.

A study in 1973 in Verona, Italy gave SAM-e to 20 depressed patients for 15 days; 10 were given only placebos. Using appropriate testing tools, the study found that the SAM-e group showed some improvements from depressive moods, including attitude toward work, among others. The researchers reported the rapid success of SAM-e in treating depressive symptoms as having occurred in as few as 4 to 7 days—and with no side effects. The SAM-e group showed reduced scores on the Hamilton Depression and Anxiety Rating Scales and also Zung's self-rating scale for depression when compared with TENS (transcutaneous electrical nerve stimulation) treatments.

Some people have blamed biochemical imbalances, such as low levels of serotonin, for fibromyalgia depressive moods. Lack of serotonin will eventually result in lack of restorative sleep, poor muscle micro-trauma repair and more pain.

A comparison of the effects of SAM-e with those of regular antidepressants shows the following:

- SAM-e is quicker, showing results in as few as 4 to 7 days;
- SAM-e leaves no real side effects, even in large doses;

- SAM-e is non-toxic;
- SAM-e need not be discontinued, since older persons may need to supplement anyway.

SAM-E and Muscle Pain and Tender Points

Clinical trials involving over 22,000 patients all found SAM-e as effective in relieving muscle pain as NSAIDs (non-steroidal anti-inflammatory drugs), without leaving their side effects. A recent news report indicated that as many as 103,000 patients are hospitalized annually due to the serious gastric side effects of NSAIDs. About 16,500 fatalities are reported to have resulted from these serious gastric side effects.

A study reported in *Current Therapeutic Research* by Dr. P. DiBenedetto and colleagues compared SAM-e with TENS (transcutaneous electrical nerve stimulation) on 30 fibromyalgia patients over a 6-week period. In the study, 15 patients each received a 200 mg injection of SAM-e in the morning and a 200 mg tablet at noon and in the evening. Another 15 persons received only TENS units to wear. All were tested using appropriate scales at the end of study. The study found that SAM-e, when compared with TENS usage, reduced more tender points and had a significant beneficial effect on symptoms such as pain and fatigue.

Another process through which SAM-e exerts its effects on pain is the process called aminopropylation. It is a process in which the polyamines spermidine and spermine are formed. These have important roles in tissue and cell growth. Another by-product of this process is a compound called methyl-thioadenosine (MTA), which is known to be a player in the body's regulation of pain and inflammatory processes.

SAM-E and Migraine Headaches

According to SAM-e researcher Dr. Dallas Clouatre, SAM-e is known to have beneficial effects for the relief of migraine headaches. According to Dr. Clouatre, the mechanism by which

SAM-e is effective is not properly known, but may be due to an improvement in membrane fluidity and catecholamine balance regulation.

SAM-e's Role in Controlling System Levels of Toxins, Oxidants, Histamine and Allergens

SAM-e is able to regulate levels of toxins and other harmful metabolites in the system by influencing the production of the body's primary antioxidant and free-radical scavenger called glutathione. Free radicals are byproducts of glycolysis that are harmful to the body and may be involved with the problem of fibromyalgia. Another antioxidant produced in association with SAM-e is taurin. The process resulting in taurin's production is known as transsulfuration.

Asthma, allergies and other disease conditions, including fibromyalgia, may be worsened or maintained by histamines in the body. Histamine is set off when organs that are exposed to the environment, like skin and the respiratory tract, come in contact with substances called allergens. The body regulates the amount of histamine in the body through an enzyme called histamine N-methyltransferase (HMT). This enzyme, according to biochemist Dr. Cooney, requires SAM-e as a methyl donor. This makes SAM-e an important player in histamine level regulation.

Other Recent Scientific Studies on the Effects of SAM-e on Fibromyalgia

Italy 1987

Evaluation of SAM-e in primary fibromyalgia. A double-blind crossover study. Conducted by Dr. A. Tavoni and associates.

Procedure: 17 people with fibromyalgia took part in a scientific investigiation in which each group receives one form of treatment before "crossing over" to get another type. Group A received 200 mg of SAM-e daily and orally, while Group B received what looked like SAM-e but was not (placebo). After 21 days both groups stopped taking anything. They were given

14 days to cool off. Why? So that whatever each group took would wear off.

Then after 14 days, the groups switched places. When the results were tallied, the researchers found a significant amount of improvement in the moods and fewer numbers of painful sites and tender points in the SAM-e groups (Group A) than the placebo groups (Group B). Because of this, those doctors decided that SAM-e is indeed effective in treating primary fibromyalgia.

Denmark 1991

Oral SAM-e in primary fibromyalgia. Double-blind clinical evaluation. Conducted by Dr. Jacobsen and associates. Reported in the *Scandinavian Journal of Rheumatology.*

Procedure: 44 fibromyalgia patients participated. Twenty received 800 mg of SAM-e daily and orally. The other group of 20 received just placebo. It is called double-blind because nobody knew what they actually received—SAM-e or a tablet that looked like SAM-e but was not. After the 6-week study, the investigators reported an improvement in fibromyalgia symptoms of fatigue, pain, morning stiffness and mood in the SAM-e group when compared to placebo group.

Italy 1994

Primary fibromyalgia is responsive to SAM-e. Conducted by Drs. Grassetto and Varotto. Reported in Current Therapeutic Research.

Procedure: 47 fibromyalgia patients were treated with 200 mg of SAM-e given intramuscularly once daily and 400 mg orally twice (800 mg) daily for 6 weeks. Researchers found at the end of study that SAM-e had improved participants' fibromyalgia symptoms of tender points, depressive moods and anxiety. The overall verdict on SAM-e's performance was that it was an effective remedy for depressed moods, pain and general well-being. And since poor sleep is a by-product of pain, SAM-e would also be beneficial in improving sleep quality.

United States 1994

SAM-e in Sjögren's syndrome and fibromyalgia.

Procedure: 30 patients with Sjögren's syndrome, fibromyalgia or both were treated with 200 mg of SAM-e given by intramuscular injection. All patients showed some improvements in their depression and for the fibromyalgia-only participants, there was a significant improvement and reduction in number of painful sites.

CHAPTER 11

~

Other Uses of SAM-e

As we have already discussed, SAM-e is able to affect and modulate several of our bodies' metabolic processes due to its readiness to donate its reactive methyl group to several receptor molecules to form new compounds. SAM-e, through methylation, transsulfuration and a host of other lesser-known processes, is able to maintain our bodies in optimal health. It can also repair the damage done and alleviate symptoms of other disease states such as

- Osteoarthritis;
- Liver diseases;
- Brain diseases such as Parkinson's and Alzheimer's;
- Cardiovascular diseases;
- Many others.

SAM-e and Osteoarthritis

Osteoarthritis is a degenerative joint disease that affects millions of Americans. It attacks the normally smooth joint surfaces of our bones. Cracks and fissures develop. Weight-bearing stresses worsen the condition. In time, the synovial fluid, which lubricates the joint surfaces, dries up or leaks into the fissures or cracks, and then into the bones. Gradually blood vessels grow out of these cracks and into the gaps in the joints, which they occlude, or block. Osteophytes or bony outgrowths form and end up restricting joint motion. By this time, the joint is usually swollen and movement is very painful.

The usual treatment of choice is NSAIDs—non-steroidal anti-inflammatory drugs—and other pain medications. These drugs have been known to cause adverse reactions such as protein breakdown and can inhibit cartilage formation and proteoglycan synthesis. Other problems associated with long-term use of NSAIDs include serious gastric problems.

SAM-e provides comparable relief to arthritis pain when compared to NSAIDs, but without any side effects. Also, SAM-e appears to promote the generation of native proteoglycan synthesis, important factors in cartilage repair.

Additionally, SAM-e may provide gastric cytoprotection against aspirin-induced hemorrhagic erosions, probably due to its ability to assist in glutathione production and its ability to protect the intestinal lining from the attacks of toxins.

SAM-e and the Liver

The liver is one of the most important and largest organs in the body. It controls processes that help sustain life; processes fats, removes toxins, produces the all-important bile. SAM-e is known to assist in many of the liver's functions and protects it from harmful toxins. SAM-e, for example, through methylation, converts phosphatidylethanolamine into phosphatidylcholine, a useful lipotropic. (A lipotropic is an agent which prevents the excessive accumulation of fat in the liver.)

In liver cirrhosis, an essential enzyme for SAM-e's product may be lacking. The disease appears to restrict "SAM-e synthetase," which results in impaired SAM-e production. Consequently, methionine, the building block of SAM-e, is not utilized. High quantities of this substance can become harmful to the liver. Because of this problem, it would be a good idea to supplement with pharmaceutical SAM-e, thereby bypassing this production impasse. This would enable SAM-e to continue to function in the liver. SAM-e is important in the liver's ability to make bile salts. Without bile salts, the liver becomes unable to digest fats. Consequently, others of its functions are stalled.

SAM-e and Brain Diseases like Parkinson's and Alzheimer's

As part of the aging process, there is a decline in the process of methylation in the brain. This decline may have some implications with the disease progress of Parkinson's and Alzheimer's.

Parkinson's disease is a degenerative problem affecting an area of the mid-brain known as the substantia nigra. This is an area whose job is to produce dopamine, which is a very important neurotransmitter. SAM-e's role in Parkinson's disease is not very clear. Actually, some people believe that high levels of SAM-e may be detrimental for this condition.

In the case of Alzheimer's, a progressive diminishing of cognitive functions occurs in areas of short-term memory. Patients have spatial problems and an inability to remember things or persons. They can sometimes behave in inappropriate or even bizarre manners.

SAM-e's role in Alzheimer's is not well known by the research community. What they do know, however, is that SAM-e levels are severely decreased in these patients as compared to the levels of SAM-e in unaffected subjects. Some interpret this as a supply and demand situation, i.e., excessive need for SAM-e, which the aging brain is unable to supply. This argument is buttressed by the fact that some memory function improvements can be achieved with SAM-e supplementation in some cases.

SAM-e and Cardiovascular Diseases

Cardiovascular disease affects the blood vessels and the coronary arteries of the heart. The most common of such heart conditions is atherosclerosis. This is the blocking of the arteries by a combination of fatty substances, cholesterol and other wastes. A person is said to suffer a heart attack when the occlusion of a heart artery shuts off blood supply to the heart. Common risk factors include cigarette smoking, high cholesterol levels, diabetes and inactivity.

64

SAM-e's role in heart disease involves controlling the levels of homocysteine, a well-known culprit in heart diseases. Homocysteine allegedly promotes the accumulation of waste in the inner lining of blood vessels by irritating of those linings. Homocysteine can also prevent the vessels from dilating sufficiently. In a normal system, homocysteine is a by-product of methylation and transsulfuration. Deficiencies of nutrients like folic acid, Vitamin B_{12} and Vitamin B_6 have been known to impair normal methylation and transsulfurization processes. So these supplements should be taken along with SAM-e.

CHAPTER 12

~

How to Take SAM-e
for Fibromyalgia

Make Sure you Buy the Right SAM-e

I have heard some people complain that SAM-e didn't seem to work for them even after one week of taking it. There are various reasons possible for this. Questions you can ask yourself about the SAM-e you are taking are:

- *Did you take SAM-e at all?* SAM-e is so unstable that if not packaged and stored properly, its potency will quickly disappear.

- *Was your SAM-e up to standard?* Were you sure that what was claimed on the label was actually what was inside the bottle? Remember the FDA does not regulate the manufacture and distribution of SAM-e as it does prescription drugs. So you really are responsible for making sure you purchase the right SAM-e.

- *Did you take the appropriate dosage of SAM-e?* And how did you take it? With vodka? On an empty or full stomach? These things do matter a lot.

Dosage would depend on your condition and its severity. But SAM-e is quite safe. Your main limitation, I suspect, might be the size of your wallet. Presently, SAM-e is very expensive.

Some of What is Known
about Pharmaceutical Grade SAM-e

Absorption

The amount of SAM-e that eventually enters your blood-stream and the length of time it takes to get there depends on the following factors:

- Its ability to remain intact until it reaches your blood-stream;

- How fast the liver metabolizes it and how quickly your kidneys excrete it;

- The dosage—the higher the dosage, the greater its staying power.

The length of time it takes a certain quantity of SAM-e to get to half of its original quantity in the blood is known as its half-life. That is, if it takes 3 hours for 200 mg of SAM-e to get to 100 mg, the half-life is 3 hours. Researchers have put SAM-e's half-life to about 101 minutes for a dosage of 500 mg.

The rate of SAM-e absorption is fastest with intravenous administration. The slowest is oral administration. But the advantage of oral administration is that the supplement will act for a longer period. The optimal absorption of SAM-e is achieved in the intestines—*not* in the stomach. So to allow it to get past the stomach's digestive environment, SAM-e should be taken in an *enteric-coated* form. SAM-e is best absorbed when taken on an empty stomach.

Toxicity

There is no evidence of its toxicity in humans. In rats, an ingestion of 1200 mg per kg of body weight daily for about 30 days did not produce any adverse symptoms, and it did not upset the digestive system. This is perhaps one of the reasons SAM-e should be preferred over NSAIDs, especially in osteoporosis. In osteoporosis, unlike the NSAIDs, which are notorious for impeding cartilage damage repair, SAM-e actually helps produce a cartilage-repairing protein called proteoglycan.

Dosage

Some experts recommend a dosage of between 200 mg and 400 mg of enteric-coated SAM-e two times a day. That is a total of up to 800 mg daily.

Possible Side Effects

There are not many. Some clinical studies have reported some mild gastrointestinal upsets and nausea in some people, particularly in those on very high doses. If this becomes a problem for you, start with a small dosage and progress until you achieve your own optimal dosage. You can also consume a large daily dosage by taking small single dosages spread throughout the day.

Contraindications

Methionine may be harmful to menopausal and post-menopausal women. Please use with care, paying attention to your body's reaction, if any. If you have manic psychological illness, please discuss with your psychiatrist before using SAM-e. Some clinical studies suggest SAM-e may be contraindicated for manic-depressive states.

Optimal Dosage Recommendation

This is only a guideline. Talk to your doctor, especially if you plan to stop your addictive medications. I am not aware of any reported drug interaction problems with SAM-e.

For Fibromyalgia with Depressive Moods

Take 400 mg of SAM-e 3 to 4 times daily (maximum 1600 mg)

Start with 200 mg 2 times daily for day #1

Increase to 400 mg 2 times daily by day #3

Increase to 400 mg 3 times daily by day #10

Reach a maximum dosage of 400 mg 4 times daily after 20 days and continue as needed.

As you get better, decrease to a daily maintenance of 800 mg, divided into two doses.

Osteoarthritis

Use the same method as outlined for fibromyalgia, but instead, max out at 400 mg 3 times daily on day #10, and continue at that dosage for another 10 days or more as needed. After about one month at maximum dosage, you might want to reduce to a maintenance dose of 200 mg 2 times daily.

Liver Disorders

200 mg to 400 mg 2 to 3 times daily

Migraine Headaches

200 mg to 400 mg 2 to 3 times daily

Depression

Use same exact method as recommended for fibromyalgia with depressive symptoms.

SAM-e for Regular Supplementation

For use to boost your body's methylation system, 200 mg 2 to 3 times daily might be sufficient.

~

CHAPTER 13

Ideas about How to Safely Come Off Your Current Addictive Medications

What to Do About Withdrawal Symptoms

Your life with fibromyalgia syndrome may be likened to a ship caught in a stormy sea–the sea of pain—and you are supposed to be the captain. But are you really the captain of your life or have you given over command to someone else? Perhaps your doctor? Too much medication may have immobilized the captain. It is very important that you remain in charge. After all, it is still *your* life, no one else's.

Some people buy into some myths about our country's current healthcare situation, such as:

- My doctor knows best; whatever he prescribes is fine.

- If the FDA approved it, it must be good.

- I heard it on TV, many people are taking it, therefore, it must be good.

All the above are false assumptions. Your doctor may mean well, but he is only a pawn within the managed care game. Besides, he may be the product of a conventional mindset about treating fibromyalgia symptoms, while ignoring the underlying problems, like lifestyle options and choices, bad habits, relationship issues, spirituality and a host of other predisposing factors. Some of these factors were not typically taught in basic medical training, although that problem may now be changing now with the current demand for and fascination with alternative or integrative medicine.

The second myth concerns the FDA and its drug approval process. The FDA may not be as impartial a watchdog as it is purported to be. Powerful drug companies and other interest groups may be holding the leash from behind the scenes.

The drug companies court medical students right up to graduation and beyond with public relation gifts and incentive offers. Doctors' offices are full of public relations items and drug samples. The drug companies fund medical studies and sponsor seminars that doctors must attend in order to maintain their certifications. They keep medical research journals in print by maintaining the huge advertisement budgets they establish.

One way or the other they try to influence what is being published. Recently, a drug company threatened to pull its enormous advertising account with a reputable medical journal simply because a study that proved detrimental to one of its products had been published in that journal.

Furthermore, TV talk shows may not be the citadel of wisdom some people think they are. This is because the producer's main concern is sensationalism. Every program is about ratings and turning huge profits. A quick fix for the current celebrated human problem is customarily touted as something revolutionary—perhaps a new pill or treatment of some kind. But there are no quick fixes. Our lifestyles are often products of lifelong lists of bad choices. Solutions to this type of struggle take time.

Sometimes medications are necessary, but we must watch out for ourselves. Medications carry with them adverse reactions, addiction problems, withdrawal reaction problems, drug interaction problems and so many other problems. So-called beneficial medications cause as many as 140,000 fatalities annually. We ought to reconsider our quick fix pill-popping mindset and consider altering our lifestyles.

Alternatives to Antidepressants

A common sense approach to avoiding antidepressant medication might include:

- Learning to cope with stress and tension;
- Learning and practicing "Muscle Tension Relaxation Technique" (which I will explain later);
- Organizing and managing your life better;
- Controlling your worry and anxiety before it controls you;
- Building up self-confidence and self-esteem;
- Establishing a restorative sleep hygiene;
- Confronting your nagging fears;
- Learning to be more assertive;
- Letting your friends and relatives know your limitations and boundaries;
- Resolving relationship problems quickly, forgiving others and moving on;
- Letting go of the past;
- Staying focused and keeping things in proper perspective;
- Above all, pray as if everything depends on God, and act as if everything depends on you.

Ideas on How to Come Off or Decrease the Dosage of your Addictive Medications

According to specialists in this field like Drs. Peter Breggin and David Cohen, the best and most sensible method is a *gradual and well-planned one.* According to these experts, "regardless of the drug you are using and the problems it may have created in your life, a well-planned, gradual withdrawal has the best chance to succeed." On the other hand, an unplanned on-the-spur-of-the-moment decision could only cause more problems and frustration.

It is crucial that you are confident in what you plan to do. Place before you always the many benefits you are hoping to achieve. List the difficulties you might encounter and expect them. Expect possible relapses. Relapses are okay; you can always try again.

Find a psychiatrist who believes in what you plan to do, and is willing to support you. Similarly, keep company with people who are likely to encourage you in your resolution. But expect that some people will be negative about it. If it didn't work for them, they will say, it won't work for you. Don't let their fears and lack of self-confidence rub off on you. But whatever happens, be in control of the situation; it is still your body and your life.

Remember, the adverse reactions you may encounter do not mean you "really need this medication." They indicate what is called "withdrawal reactions." Don't be discouraged.

Pray. God, they say, helps those who help themselves. Find a support group of relatives and friends. Find a supporter willing to speak with you often. Involve your spouse and family members. The will and enthusiasm to live fully and to take back your life from fibromyalgia will soon rub off on those around you, and they will appreciate you more. Check out the information super highway–the Internet—for encouraging websites.

A Step-by-Step Gradual Drug Withdrawal Plan

Step 1: Stabilize your dosage by taking the same amount at the same time.

Step 2: Choose a gradual stepwise method. Maybe reduce the dosage by 10% or any other amount you are comfortable with. You may start with the SAM-e program simultaneously to coincide with this. This would cushion the normal withdrawal reactions.

In the 10% technique, the dosage is decreased in ten steps, 10% at a time. You may divide the final 10% into smaller doses.

The duration of each step depends on the length of time you've been on that particular medication. This is the Law of

Habit at play. It took some time building an addiction; dismantling that habit also takes time. In general, it varies from weeks to months. You are in charge here. Make a plan and stick with it; at the same time expand your alternative medicine strategies.

For example, if you are taking 150 mg of an antidepressant, your first cutback (decrease) would be 15 mg. Perform the next eight 15 mg cuts, then you can subdivide the last or tenth 15 mg into smaller cutbacks, possibly of 5 mg each, if you prefer. Stay on each step for one week to ten days. The last step is usually the toughest; that is why you might have to subdivide it.

What to Do about Withdrawal Reactions

1. It is hoped that supplementing with SAM-e will alleviate withdrawal symptoms significantly.

2. Depending on how long you've been on medication, you might have to do very small cutbacks, even less than 10%, and remain within each range, or step, for a longer period.

3. If you are on several drugs, plan to stop one at a time. Start with the heavy ones, i.e., if you are taking one to relieve the side effects of the other, then remove the side effect medication later.

4. You may have to "cool off" for a long time after going to a lower dosage. Adjust to the reactions before decreasing to the next step, but try not to despair or discard the whole idea. You have one life to live. You will not have another chance. Think of all those who love you and need you to be strong and together. For the Christian believer, the words of Christ to Paul the apostle suffices: "My grace is sufficient for you." You have only to pray to tap into this reservoir of strength.

PART 4

Other Drug-Free Fibromyalgia Relief and Self-Care Strategies

CHAPTER 14

~

How to Manage Stress
and Muscle Tension

What Are Stress and Muscle Tension?

Stress

Life is naturally stressful. Our bodies are made up of chemicals and hormones that are constantly at war with each other. We live in a high-tech and high-pressure society, which is a maelstrom of all kinds of stressors. We can't always get what we want. We clutter our lives with things we don't need. Then, too, we have fragile egos that get in the way of meaningful relationships. We get caught up in bad habits that kill us gradually. The changes we can make, we are reluctant to make; the ones we can't, we worry needlessly over. We entertain irrational fears over things we can't control. So, we are enveloped by stressors, which gradually master our lives.

Science defines "acute stress" as a reaction to an immediate danger. This is also called the "fight or flight" response. What this means in layman's terms is that nature automatically prepares us to face danger. Our hearts beat faster and pump more blood and oxygen to the muscles where they might be needed to effect an escape or to put up a fight. Many other things happen within our bodies. This beneficial, protective reaction can become habitual. When this happens, our bodies readjust in a very wrong way. A sense of tension—or continuous fight or flight response—resides in our subconscious and continually feed our senses with undesirable stimuli. Our tension senses become acute, so every little harmless event puts our bodies on "red alert." Somehow, the physiological changes that occur when we are faced with a threat no longer return to normal once the threat has passed. This situation is known as *residual tension*.

Muscle Tension

There are two connotations to the term "muscle tension."

1. Muscle fibers are contracting needlessly, even when subject is at rest; and

2. There is a constant sense of tension as muscles remain in a shortened position and do not relax.

The following are some clinical indications of a state of muscle tension:

- Irregular and shallow breathing;
- Your mind is as busy as a beehive when you are supposed to be sleeping;
- Your brow frowns and your eyelids move uncontrollably;
- Any little thing startles you;
- Spasm of the smooth muscles of the alimentary canal;
- You can't sleep at night; you jerk and toss around.

What are the Noticeable Signs of Stress?

- You get upset easily;
- You worry too much;
- You forget things and you can't concentrate;
- You procrastinate;
- You can't seem to keep appointments or manage your time well;
- You start taking tranquilizers;
- Because of poor sleep quality, your muscles are always sore.

The Short-Term Effects of Stress, i.e., the "Fight or Flight" Response

Each stressful episode starts a chain reaction in your system:

- Large quantities of epinephrine are released into your bloodstream;
- Your heart beats faster;
- Your blood pressure rises;
- Your breathing becomes faster and shallow;
- Your metabolic rate escalates;
- Muscle tension rises with increased lactic acid;
- Your blood gets re-routed to your muscles away from the digestive system, resulting in an imbalance in the digestive juices;
- The digestive juices start chopping away at your stomach lining causing ulcers;
- Cortisol decreases your immune system, so you easily get sick and have frequent flu and fevers.

The Long-Term Effects of Stress

If you do nothing about how you react to stress and you live an habitual life of stress and tension, gradually, your body adjusts and produces more serious symptoms like:

- High blood pressure;
- Frequent headaches;
- Sleep problems;
- Irritability;
- High cholesterol levels, which eventually will clog your arteries;
- Struggling to catch your breath with little exertion;
- Palpitations of the heart; perhaps development of abnormal heart rhythms;

- Muscle and back pain due to decreased blood flow of nutrients and oxygen, and accumulation of metabolites like lactic acid;
- Nausea caused by gastric acid production imbalance;
- Ulcers;
- Frequent illnesses due to production of too much cortisol, which weakens your immune system;
- Depressive moods.

Physiological Relaxation

What Is Relaxation?

Now that we understand the serious problems caused by stress, we must now turn our attention to its exact opposite—relaxation. Relaxation provokes opposite physiological reactions to those brought about by stress. Some of these include:

- Decreased epinephrine in the blood. This leads to a lowering of blood pressures, thereby exerting less stress on the cardiovascular system.
- Less clogging of arteries due to reduced blood sugar and cholesterol. Risk of heart attack is reduced significantly.
- Slower and deeper breathing. More oxygen and nutrients get to the brain and the muscles. This improves metabolic rate.
- Improved quality of sleep, allowing the secretion of repairing hormones from the pituitary gland.
- Improved digestion. Absence of ulcers allows you to enjoy all kinds of food.
- The immune system remaining in top shape; you become less prone to illnesses.

The overall effect of relaxation is a regular state of serenity, with increased alertness and spontaneity. So the state of relaxation is a very desirable one, especially for the fibromyalgia sufferer.

But it doesn't come easily. For most people in our society, it is a skill that must be learned. Once learned and practiced regularly, however, relaxation becomes second nature. This science of relaxation is called "Progressive Muscle Relaxation." Once you master the art of relaxation, you won't ever need tranquilizers to calm down. And you will learn to relax beyond the residual tension state.

What Happens in "Physiological" Relaxation?

Physiological relaxation is the forerunner or prerequisite to complete physical relaxation. Achieving physiological relaxation is evidenced physically by:

- A complete absence of muscle contraction, in which muscle fibers remain in a lengthened position;

- The big skeletal muscles becoming limp;

- Rates of impulse firing and excitability of nerves becoming reduced or even inactive.

Progressive Relaxation Technique

Although there are many types of progressive relaxation techniques, it is best to learn and master just one technique. It doesn't really matter how you become relaxed—just *that* you become relaxed. The concept of progressive relaxation technique was first described as a science by Dr. Edmund Jacobson in 1908, followed by other investigators of this phenomenon, including Dr. Herbert Benson. In 1970, Dr. Benson wrote his definitive book on the subject called *The Relaxation Response*. The "relaxation response" is basically the opposite of the "fight or flight" response to a threat or stressful event.

How Much Time Do You Need?

Researchers have found that a 20-minute practice each day is very beneficial to both physical and mental health.

What You Need to Induce a Relaxation Response

- A quiet environment;
- A comfortable position;
- A point of focus;
- A passive attitude;

Most people always manage to make time for things that they consider important, like catching their favorite talk show, for instance. We know time can be reserved for special things every day, so try to make time for relaxation daily—it's an extremely important ingredient to your overall health. It may very well make the difference between life and death. And it will certainly improve and prolong your life.

Breathing Exercise

Some of the benefits of *biofeedback therapy* include helping you become aware of subtle muscle activity that you are not ordinarily conscious of. (In biofeedback therapy, electrodes or probes are used to connect a patient to a "feedback" machine that monitors subtle physical changes. A patient, by responding to signals, or "feedback" from this device, learns to self-regulate her body functions like breathing.) Once you become aware of such muscle activity, you can use your muscles better. Also, this type of therapy teaches you breathing skills, which encourage muscle tension release and physiologic quieting.

Improper and shallow breathing habits prevent your muscles from getting the oxygen and nutrients they need. It is therefore important to re-learn how to breathe properly. A common method is called "diaphragmatic breathing technique."

Figure 14-1: Diaphragmatic Breathing Technique

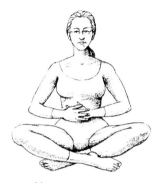

A. Sit comfortably as shown. Place both of your hands on your stomach just below the rib cage. Breathe in gradually and deeply through the nose. Allow your diaphragm to move down and flatten as your stomach moves forward pushing out your hands. Feel your fingers fan out.

B. Hold your breath for about 5 seconds and gradually breathe out through the nose. Feel your diaphragm relax and your stomach sink. Try to let out as much air as possible.

C. Repeat this procedure 3 to 4 times. Focus your mind on this exercise; avoid all distractions. Your chest is supposed to remain still during this exercise. If it moves, you may be doing it incorrectly.

D. Practice with your spouse (see below). Everybody needs it to relax completely; your spouse probably needs it more than you do! Besides, it is a nice way of communicating and getting involved.

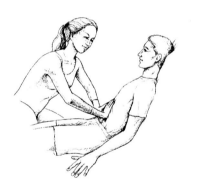

Figure 14-2: Two-Person Breathing Technique

Assume position as in Figure 14-2. Place your hands in the shape of a "V" below your spouse's rib cage. Ask him or her to breathe in slowly, allowing the stomach to rise. Make sure your spouse's chest is not moving. Feel his or her stomach pushing out your hands. Then ask your spouse to slowly let out air through the nose. Repeat 3 to 4 times. Switch positions and repeat the procedure.

Progressive Muscle Relaxation Technique

Remember, you will need the following:

- A quiet environment;
- A comfortable position;
- A point of focus;
- A passive attitude.

Step 1. Quiet environment

This is difficult to find or arrange when you have children. But you must find one. Be creative; negotiate if you must. Place "do not disturb" signs on doors; sneak down to the basement. Just find the space and do it!

Step 2. A comfortable position

Depending on what your goal is, assume position of figure 14-3 (lying down) if you intend to drift off, or position of figure 14-4 (sitting or reclining). You can also sit straight (as in figure 14-1) with a straight spine or you can sit cross-legged.

Step 3. A point of focus

Choose a special word or phrase and repeat it throughout the session. This is very similar to the Christian form of meditation called the "Jesus Prayer" and in fact is used as a relaxation prayer. It goes like this: "Jesus, Son of the living God, have mercy on me, a sinner," or "The Lord is my Shepherd, I shall not want." You can practice with eyes either open or closed. If open, try to focus on some object, otherwise your mind will wander with your eyes.

Step 4. A passive attitude

Let it happen. Right now, in this place and time, you don't care about anything. Don't worry about any distracting thoughts; this is normal. Gently turn about your attention to your point of focus.

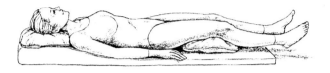

Figure 14-3: Relaxation Position: Lying Down
   Place pillows under the head and knees, lay arms loosely at your sides with the palms face down on the mattress. You should feel completely relaxed. This position is called "the neutral position." Tension is zero.

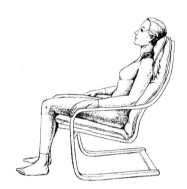

Figure 14-4: Relaxation Position: Sitting Down
   Sit comfortably in a high-backed chair that supports your head and whole spine. Place both arms tension-free on the armrests as shown.

Step 5. Progressive muscle relaxation

There are several methods. The best is whichever suits your personality. The point is to relax. You can't relax unless you can identify the feeling of tension. Then, you strive for the opposite feeling. So, to begin, you need to forcefully contract each group of large skeletal muscles before you attempt to relax them. If you are experiencing pain and are worried that contracting your muscles will exacerbate the problem, then do not contract them. This step is not necessary for you, because you already know what tension is. Just relax consciously, as if you are deflating an inflated object. The part of the body with which you start is not really important, although it is advisable to end with the head. Below is my regimen.

A. *Feet and toes:* Start with the toes and move up. Crunch your toes and rotate your feet about your ankles, then release.

B. *Leg muscles:* Move your ankles completely up and down, hold and release.

C. *Thigh muscles:* If you are lying down, press down the back of your knee on the pillow or a rolled towel and squeeze your thighs or quads. Hold and release. If sitting, hook your feet under something and try to raise it while squeezing thighs; hold and release.

D. *Buttocks:* Squeeze them, hold and release.

E. *Stomach:* Pull it in, hold and release.

F. *Shoulders and back:* Shrug shoulders and pull them backward, hold and release. Arch the back, hold and release.

G. *Neck muscles:* If you are sitting, place both hands behind your head and push head backwards against your hands' resistance, hold and then release.

If you are lying, stiffen the muscles of the neck, hold and then release.

H. *Arms and hands:* Flex (show off) your biceps, i.e., bend your elbows, hold and release. Make a tight fist, hold and release.

I. *Head and facial muscles:* Wrinkle your forehead, hold and release. Frown deeply, hold and release. Move from pursing your lips to a wide grin, repeat and release.

J. *Eyes:* Close the eyes tightly. Look up while maintaining your head position, then relax the eyes. Look down and repeat procedure. Relaxing the eyes—brows or lids— needs a lot of practice. If you are not able to relax the eyes, try to do so in conjunction with relaxing the right arm.

General Comments

Muscle relaxation can be interspersed with the breathing exercise.

1. Hold tension for about 10 to 15 seconds.

2. Release in three steps.

3. You can breathe in as you contract and hold, and breathe out as you release.

   - Rest for about 1 minute or more in between muscle groups.

   - Tense and release only one group of muscles at a time, keeping the rest of your body perfectly still and relaxed.

Enhancements to Progressive Muscle Relaxation

Certain enhancements to the regimen can make it more a valuable and more pleasant experience.

Visualization

Create your favorite picture of peace and serenity in your mind, and stay there. If your worries come up again, gently notice them and go back to your peaceful place.

Aromatherapy

You can light your favorite aromatic candle and put on gentle relaxation music or sound like singing birds, gentle rainfall, etc.

Dealing with Impediments to Relaxation

Worrying

Worry, in general, is a stream of thoughts of fear that an event might occur. Your mind runs free like a wild horse that you must tame. Set aside a worry-time, when you can dwell on finding resolutions to the source of worry.

I personally like to actually list strategies to prevent the event from occurring, then I reconcile myself to the worst case scenario—that it may happen. I even make contingency plans, in case it does happen. The ones I can't do anything about, I don't worry about. My religious faith assures me that a loving God is still in charge of His creation, in spite of the seeming chaos.

Anger and Resentment

Anger actually hurts the angry person. It can cause serious health complications, like heart disease and ulcers. Most of the time, anger cannot be controlled. It may be an indication that we are stressed, and it is time to take a break.

If your anger or resentment has risen to any of the following stages, it is important for you to address it:

- It is habitually on your mind and upsetting your life.
- It makes you abusive towards others.
- It is hurting your relationship with family members.

Quick Solutions to Anger

1. Acknowledge that you are angry. If you don't, it will never go away.

2. Tame your mind and force it to dwell on happy thoughts.

3. Rationalize your anger. Perhaps you are over-reacting and may need to cool off.

4. Identify your source of anger. Learn to delay responding to someone's annoying remarks. Count to ten mentally. Be in control of your responses and emotions. Often, silence is the best answer, they say.

5. Learn to listen to the other person. You might learn something that will be to your advantage. Try to see things sometimes from the other person's perspective and be firm and assertive when you must, but do so kindly.

Relationships

It is the bed you make that you lie on. If you put rocks in yours, you will either have to remove them or lie on top of them, but they will continue to hurt you until you *do* remove them. No one can help you with this. If you choose to move to another bed, pretty soon you'll come to realize that most beds are basically the same. Then you will have to start all over learning how to lie on this new one. So it makes a lot of sense to take care of the old one you are used to.

The point is that little unresolved relationship issues can quickly add up and get out of hand. Move away from too much self-preoccupation and realize that your spouse, for example, has feelings, too. Appreciate his or her efforts to understand and support you with your life of pain. See an appropriate therapist to help you resolve difficult issues, like those involving sex. Your psychiatrist can perhaps change your antidepressants to those that do not impair libido.

Humans, they say, are social beings. You can't be alone for too long and not pay for it in mental health. You need your friends and relatives to feel valued, important and loved. A huge ego is a handicap; it is not in your best interest. Be the first to call and mend a relationship. If you want to change others, start by changing yourself.

Find a support group and attend meetings. This is an opportunity to be with people who can affect you in your current situation in a very positive way. You can learn new remedies to your health problems, or learn about other sources of help.

The Importance of Laughing

"We don't laugh because we're happy – we're happy because we laugh."   – William James, psychologist

Nothing deflates anger and sadness more quickly than laughter. If a friend or something provokes us to laughter, we soon realize the foolishness of our depressive moods. There is now a science (called humor therapy) that deals with humor and treatment of disease states. According to noted author Norman Cousins' *(Anatomy of An Illness)* discovery, 10 minutes of vigorous laughing bought him 2 hours of good sleeping without drugs or pain. Some researchers believe that laughing stimulates the release of chemical messengers in the brain known as endorphins, which are natural sedatives. After a bout of laughter, blood pressure monitoring usually shows a decrease in readings, breathing is slower and deeper and muscles more relaxed. If you don't find anything funny enough, go watch a good comedy movie. If that doesn't do it, watch yourself in a mirror and start laughing; pretty soon you will be laughing for real.

CHAPTER 15

~

Fibromyalgia Exercise
and Fitness Program

Movement is a major characteristic of all living organisms. The lack of it has a very great impact on the quality of life itself. Lack of exercise, especially for a prolonged period of time, for whatever reason, has very profound effects on human cardio-vascular, neuromuscular and metabolic systems. These effects can come about very rapidly.

For over a decade, I worked with geriatric patients in nursing homes. During my time there, I was able to observe first-hand how rapidly the muscles could succumb to inactivity. Most elderly end up losing the ability to walk and, thus, independence. The adage that "if you don't use it, you'll lose it" holds very true for muscles. Some of the well-known effects of lack of exercise include:

- Low energy and work capacity due to low oxygen uptake and usage;
- Decrease in muscle size, leading to decreased strength;
- Decreased cardiac efficiency leading to a decrease in blood circulation—plasma and red blood cells—which can lead to several kinds of heart diseases;
- Decreased amount of air in the lungs;
- Increased amount of calcium excreted in urine, leading to osteoporosis and fractures.

These problems have a ripple effect as they quickly create other health complications. Having a very painful condition, like fibromyalgia, is not a good enough excuse to refrain from exercise. We must find ways to control the pain; pace ourselves, but seize all available opportunity to exercise to a target heart rate of 60% to 80% of our maximum heart rate for about 20 to 30 minutes a day, at least three times a week.

Some Scientific Investigations about Fibromyalgia and Exercise

A study to determine the effectiveness of physical training in women with fibromyalgia. Conducted by C.S. Burkhart and others and reported in the *Journal of Rheumatology*.

Ninety-nine women with fibromyalgia participated in this study and were divided into three groups. The first group received only advice on self-management, the second group received advice and physical training, while the third group served as a control only and received no advice. The results showed that those in groups one and two had significant improvements in quality of life as evidenced by a decrease in feelings of helplessness, tender points, depressive moods and physical dysfunction.

A study to determine the effects of cardiovascular fitness on fibromyalgia. Conducted by G.A. McCain, D.A. Bell and associates. Studies were reported in the *Arthritis and Rheumatology Journal*.

Forty-two patients with fibromyalgia were split into two groups and participated in this research program for 20 weeks. One group received cardiovascular fitness (CVR), the other group received only simple flexibility exercises (FLEX) that did not promote cardiovascular fitness. The exercise took place for a period of one hour, three times each week.

The results showed significant improvement in cardiovascular fitness scores in the CVR group over the FLEX group. Furthermore, the CVR group also showed significant improvements in pain threshold values.

There are several other studies that demonstrate favorably the beneficial effects of exercise and fitness training on reducing the symptoms of fibromyalgia. The major salient points to be deduced from these studies include:

- Exercise improves the ability to cope with the chronic pain associated with fibromyalgia;
- Exercise alleviates depressive moods;
- Exercise improves cardiovascular health;
- Cardiovascular fitness requires aerobic activity;
- Fibromyalgia patients can participate in aerobic, flexibility and strength training exercises without adverse effects.

According to Dr. George W. Waylonis, a professor of physical medicine and rehabilitation at Ohio State University, "The most effective treatments for fibromyalgia are exercise, over-the-counter pain medications and avoidance of stress factors." According to several clinical studies, fibromyalgia patients are generally de-conditioned. Therefore, a well-tailored exercise program composes the cornerstone of an effective treatment program.

Exercise Guidelines for Fibromyalgia

According to Dr. Russel, director of the Clinical Research Center at the University of Texas Health Science Center in San Antonio, fibromyalgia exercise and fitness programs should be started slowly, and progressed gradually according to the patient's tolerance. He points out, "Unaccustomed physical exertion can induce severe body pain and incapacitate the patient for the next several days."

- Have a medical check-up for exercise risk factors before embarking on a program. You can be at risk if you:
  - have heart problems;
  - often complain of chest pain;

– often feel faint and dizzy;

– have a history of high blood pressure.

- Select activities that you enjoy, like swimming or walking.

- Listen to your body. Find a time and place that will be suitable for your unique personality and condition. If you happen to feel more relaxed and have less pain and more energy in the evenings, by all means exercise in the evenings, as long as it is at least four hours before bedtime.

- Once you start, please be consistent, so you can gain most of the rewards of exercise.

- Exercise at your own comfortable pace. Watch out for unusual amounts of pain, breathlessness or dizziness.

- Wear weather-appropriate clothing and comfortable shoes.

- Spice up your exercise program with variety. Find exercise partners who have your level of conditioning. Working with a partner can support and motivate you.

- Set some goals that are small and achievable, and also challenge yourself. Reward yourself for your goal achievements.

- Watch out for abnormal symptoms such as chest pain or heaviness in the chest area; pronounced palpitations and breathlessness, especially with minor exertion; wheezing; nausea and faintness; numbness or too much pain. It is normal for your pulse to be faster during and after exercise, as well as to have some minor palpitations, sweating, deeper and faster breathing.

- In case of injury during exercise, perform the following first aid:

  – Protect the injured area from further assault;

  – Rest the injured area;

  – Apply a cold compress to reduce swelling if any, or stop bleeding.

  – Resume your exercise program as pain and injury permits.

How Much Exercise Should You Do?

As I mentioned earlier, listen to your body. Exercise intensity is usually a combination of how often, how hard and how long you exercise. Simple guidelines you can follow include:

• Do not continue when there is too much pain;

• Exercise about three times a week; that is, on alternate days;

• How hard? Exercise within your heart-rate zone;

• How long? Usually 20 to 30 minutes at a time.

What to Do about Constant Muscle Soreness and Pain

Muscle soreness or pain is usually due to lack of adequate blood flow and the oxygen and nutrients it carries. It is also due to a buildup of metabolites, like lactic acid.

Fibromyalgia patients are advised to take a long, warm bath before their exercise and fitness program. A warm bath promotes blood circulation and therefore sends more oxygen to the muscle tissues, which, in turn, will help flush out the metabolites.

Perhaps the best exercise program for fibromyalgia and other chronic pain patients is swimming or pool exercise activity, with the pool temperature at about 88°.

What is Your Lifestyle Activity Level?

Are you a turtle or a hare? You have a "turtle" or sedentary lifestyle if you spend most of your time engaged in the following activities:

• Frequent naps;

• Too much TV;

• Writing;

• Sewing or needlework;

• Sitting in the car, bus or train when you venture out.

You could have a "hare" or moderate lifestyle activity level if you spend significant amounts of time doing the following:

- Walking at about four miles an hour;
- Raking leaves;
- Mopping floors;
- Walking up and down stairs.

Some benefits of improving your lifestyle activity level include:

- Significant reduction to your risk of heart disease and stroke;
- Reduction of body fat, thus avoiding the complications of obesity;
- Building and preservation of your muscles, and improvement of your metabolic rate;
- A break in your stress cycle and improvement over depressive moods;
- Improvement of your self-esteem, confidence and social life;
- Improvement in your endurance and stamina, making you less prone to injury and boosting your immune system.

The Fibromyalgia Exercise and Fitness Program

The program comprises:

- Breathing Exercise
- Stretching Program
- Aerobic Exercise
- Strength Training

In order for exercise to be beneficial to you, adequate planning is essential. The more frequently you exercise, the less time you will need to achieve results. But try not to overdo things. Your exercise program ought to contain the above four types of exercise. In addition, each exercise program should start with a warm-up session and end with a cool-down session.

I encourage you to perform some type of exercise daily. You will soon get used to it and you will love it. This is one addiction that can do you a ton of good. If you choose to exercise daily, a simple plan would be to perform an alternate enjoyable activity between a stretching, aerobic or strength-training day. Please use light weights for strengthening. I advocate the use of gravity, light ankle or wrist weights, and exercise rubber bands used in physical therapy centers.

Limit strength training to not more than three times a week, initially, because your muscle fibers need some time between sessions to recover. On the activity day, you may just walk around the block or in a park.

Warm-up Session
Warm-up is a necessary pre-condition for a safe exercise program. The reasons for this are:

- It will improve your exercise performance by promoting your body's circulatory adjustment, minimizing loss of oxygen and decreasing the formation of lactic acid.

- It increases muscle core temperature, which, in turn, will improve muscle efficiency and oxygen utilization.

- It allows a quicker blood flow to your lungs.

- A warm-up session makes you less prone to exercise injuries.

A warm-up session is usually 10 minutes of stretching exercises; whole body gradual movements as in calisthenics; yoga; or running very slowly.

Cool-Down Session
Just like you need a warm-up session before exercise, you will also need a cool-down session after your exercise program. Good reasons for this include the fact that a cool-down session:

- Prevents the pooling of blood in the extremities;

- Prevents fainting by increasing blood flow to your heart and brain;
- Helps prevent cardiac complications like arrhythmias.

A cool-down session is basically the same as a warm-up session. Perform some stretching or calisthenics for approximately 5 to 8 minutes following your exercise program.

Stretching Program

Stretching is a general term used to describe a purposeful maneuver designed to elongate pathologically shortened soft tissues like muscles, thereby increasing the range of movement.

Flexibility is similar to and often used interchangeably with stretching. It is defined as the ability of a soft tissue, like a muscle, to relax and yield to a stretching force.

Our sample stretching program will include the following groups of exercises:

1. *Group A:* Hip, Trunk Rotation, Hamstring and Piriformis Muscle Stretch Program. Please study figures 15-1 to 15-9.

2. *Group B:* Neck Stretching Program. Please study figures 15-10a & b; 15-11a, b & c; 15-12a & b; 15-13a, b & c; 15-14a & b.

3. *Group C:* Therapy Ball Stretching Program:. Please study figures 15-13 to 15-23.

Group A: Hip, Trunk Rotation, Hamstring and Piriformis Muscle Stretch Program

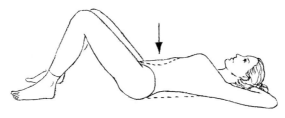

Figure 15-1: Pelvic Tilt

Place a rolled-up towel underneath your waist; press down on it while contracting your abdominal muscles and tilting your pelvis backward; hold for 5 to 10 seconds.

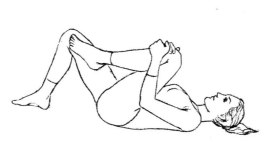

Figure 15-2: Knee to Chest

Bring each knee individually up to chest, pull and hold for 5-10 seconds; alternate.

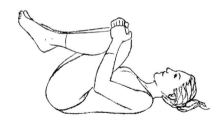

Figure 15-3: Both Knees to Chest
Repeat as in figure 15-2, but bring both knees to chest at the same time.

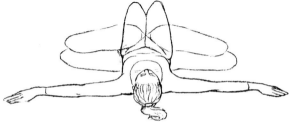

Figure 15-4: Trunk Rotation
Bend and keep knees together as shown, keeping feet on the floor. Stabilize upper trunk and rotate side to side. Hold for 5 to 10 seconds at the end of the rotation to each side.

Figure 15-5: Hamstring Stretch
Straighten your knee and stretch with both hands on the calf and hold for 5 to 10 seconds. You can also place your heel against the wall and move your buttocks towards it. (Two-joint muscles like the hamstring easily get shortened with inactivity.)

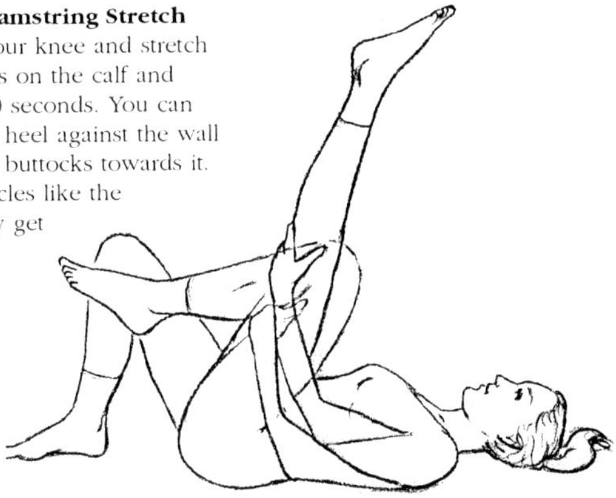

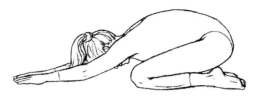

Figure 15-6: Prayer Stretch
Feel your back, shoulders and ankles stretch. Hold for 5 to 10 seconds.

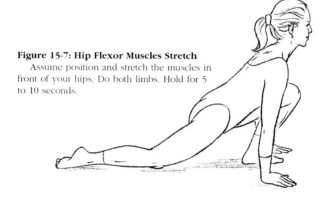

Figure 15-7: Hip Flexor Muscles Stretch
Assume position and stretch the muscles in front of your hips. Do both limbs. Hold for 5 to 10 seconds.

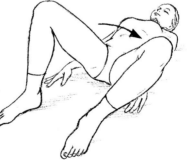

Figure 15-8:
Hip Abduction
Bend both knees, as in illustration. Keeping one limb steady, move the other completely away. Alternate between both limbs.

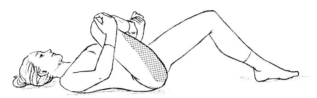

Figure 15-9: Piriformis Stretch

Bend and internally rotate your hip with both hands as shown. Hold for 5 to 10 seconds and release.

Group B: Neck Stretching Program.
Repeat Each Exercise Five Times.

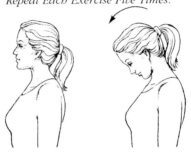

Figures 15-10a & b: Chin to Chest

Stand or sit in front of a mirror. While maintaining a good posture, slowly bring your chin toward your chest. Hold for 5 to 10 seconds and return to starting position.

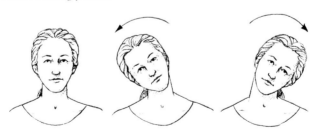

Figures 15-11a, b & c: Ear to Shoulder

Tilt your head toward right first, and then the left, as if to touch the shoulder with your ear. Hold each side for 5 to 10 seconds.

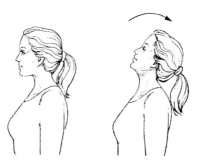

Figures 15-12a & b: Head to Back

While maintaining position of figure 15-11, move head backward. Keep your upper trunk steady and move only at the neck as you look at the ceiling. Hhold for 5 to 10 seconds and return.

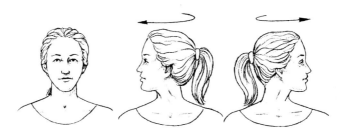

Figures 15-13a, b & c: Side Turns

While maintaining position of figure 15-12, gently turn your head to the right or left to look over your shoulder. Hold for 5 to 10 seconds and return.

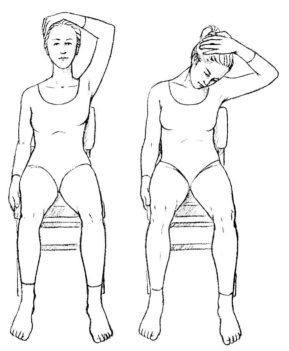

Figures 15-14a & b: Oblique Neck Muscles Stretch
Start as in position in figure 15-14a, grasp your chair for support, and grasp the back of your head with the opposite hand. Turn your head and look at the thigh opposite the hand holding onto the chair. Stretch and hold for 5 to 10 seconds. Alternate.

Group C: Therapy Ball Stretching Program

Equipment needed: Therapy or exercise ball of appropriate inflation and size.

Ball Size	Body Height
45 cm	55" to 60"
55 cm	61" to 66"
65 cm	67" to 71"
75 cm	72" to 75"
85 cm	75"+

Source of information: Thera-Bond™ Hygenic Corporation

Benefits of ball exercises: According to Caroline Corning Creager, a well-known therapy ball expert, therapy ball exercises have benefits "too numerous to list." According to Ms. Creager, some of these include:

- Muscle tension relaxation;

- Easily achieved total body stretching program;

- Improved muscle blood flow;

- Assistance in body-awareness development;

- Assistance with positive correction and spine alignment;

- Help in relief of depressive moods while energizing the body;

- Fun and entertaining for everyone in the family.

This is a low-impact exercise activity that I highly recommend to fibromyalgia sufferers. The effort of balancing on the ball elicits and exercises all postural muscles. Endurance and strength are also developed, as your muscles contract in an eccentric manner. In eccentric contraction, your muscles lengthen as they develop tension and contract to control movement produced by an external force. The therapy ball program involves the following exercises:

1. Trunk Side Stretch

2. Torso Rotational Stretch

3. Abdominal and Back Muscles Stretch (Pelvic Tilt)

4. Pelvic Circles Stretch

5. Inner Thigh Stretch

6. Piriformis Stretch

7. Calf and Hamstring Stretch

8. Side to Side Hip Stretch

9. Relaxation Bounce

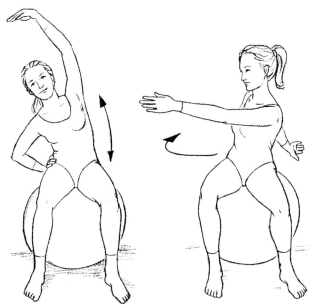

Figure 15-15:
Trunk Side Stretch

Keep hip steady with one hand. Raise the opposite arm overhead while bending at the waist until the side is fully stretched. Hold for 5 to 10 seconds. Repeat for the other side.

Figure 15-16:
Torso Rotational Stretch

Sit steady on the ball. With arms raised and extended and hips steady, rotate torso fully towards the left. Hold for 5 to 10 seconds. Repeat to the right. Note that head and upper body should move in unison.

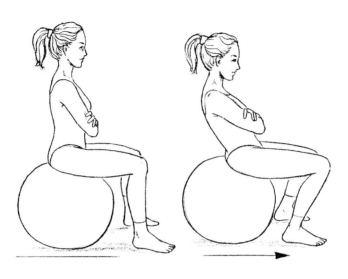

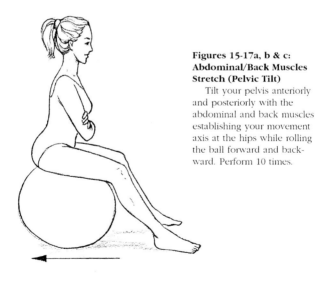

Figures 15-17a, b & c: Abdominal/Back Muscles Stretch (Pelvic Tilt)
Tilt your pelvis anteriorly and posteriorly with the abdominal and back muscles establishing your movement axis at the hips while rolling the ball forward and backward. Perform 10 times.

Figure 15-18:
Pelvic Circles Stretch
Keeping upper body steady, make circular motions with your hips on the ball. Increase circle size as tolerated. Perform 10 times.

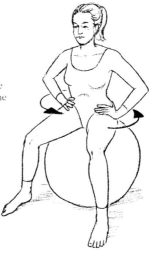

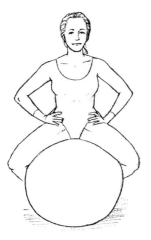

Figure 15-19:
Inner Thigh Stretch
Sit steadily on ball as shown. Place both hands on the hips and move legs behind the ball as inner thigh is stretched. Hold for 5 to 10 seconds.

Figure 15-20:
Piriformis Stretch
    Maintain your sitting balance on the ball as shown. Keep your right hand on the ball as you bend your left knee and place the ankle on your right knee. With your left hand on your left knee, gently press down and feel the stretch as your hip rotates internally. Repeat same procedure for the other limb. Hold for 5 to 10 seconds.

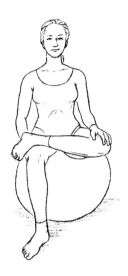

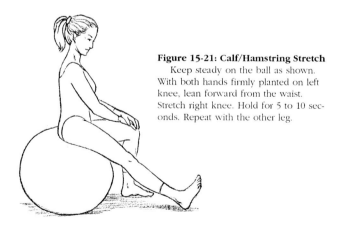

Figure 15-21: Calf/Hamstring Stretch
    Keep steady on the ball as shown. With both hands firmly planted on left knee, lean forward from the waist. Stretch right knee. Hold for 5 to 10 seconds. Repeat with the other leg.

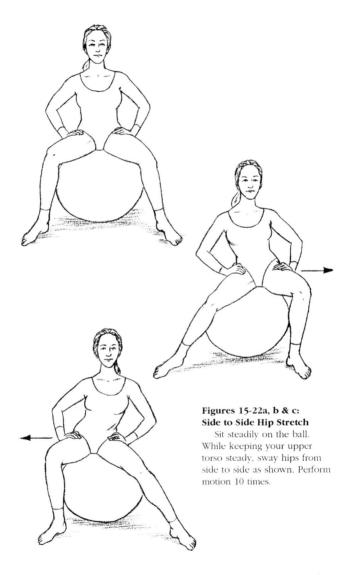

Figures 15-22a, b & c:
Side to Side Hip Stretch
   Sit steadily on the ball. While keeping your upper torso steady, sway hips from side to side as shown. Perform motion 10 times.

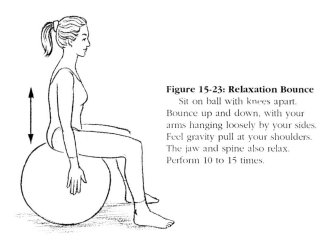

Figure 15-23: Relaxation Bounce
Sit on ball with knees apart.
Bounce up and down, with your
arms hanging loosely by your sides.
Feel gravity pull at your shoulders.
The jaw and spine also relax.
Perform 10 to 15 times.

Group D: Spinal Mobilization using an exercise foam roller

The spinal column is made up of several postural muscles and ligaments that originate and attach in oblique directions on the articulating facets. These maintain the normal "S" shaped curvature of the spine. The flexibility of the curves enables the spine to withstand ten times more axial compression forces than if it were a straight column. Balance and flexibility in the spinal system are necessary to counteract the effects of gravity and other external forces.

By rolling up and down and side to side, the tiny joints and muscles of the spine can be stretched.

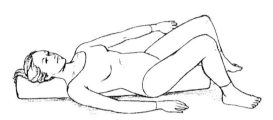

Figure 15-24a
While lying down on the foam roller, parallel with it, slowly roll from side to side. Extend one arm. Perform this 10 times.

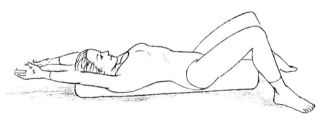

Figure 15-24b
While maintaining position in figure15-24a, slowly raise both arms up and down. Perform 10 times.

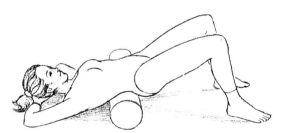

Figure 15-24c
Lie down on the roller, perpendicular to it. Cushion head with both arms. Gently and slowly roll up and down your spine. Perform 10 times.

TMJ Exercise Program

Many fibromyalgia patients have problems with their temporomandibular joints. Muscles get tight quite easily if not used often and create a lot of pain, which often radiates to the area of the face around the jaw, known as the temporomandibular joint.

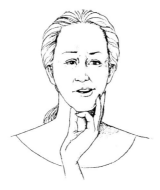

Figure 15-25: Temporomandibular Joint Exercise
Place two fingers together on the side of your jaw.
Try to resist your jaw movements with the fingers.

Some TMJ problem tips:

• Cut up your food into tiny bites so you don't have to open your mouth too wide;

• Eat very soft foods, avoid tough meat, etc.;

• Avoid chewing gum;

• Don't form the habit of biting off food with front teeth;

• If you clench and grind your teeth at night, you might consider asking your dentist for an appropriate prosthesis or bite pads.

Aerobic Exercise and Fibromyalgia

Several studies attest to the fact that aerobic and cardiovascular fitness activities are superior and more effective than any other type of exercise program in treating fibromyalgia symptoms.

Remember, exercise, especially aerobic, should be built up gradually. The eventual aim is to exercise for 20 to 30 minutes at a target heart rate of 60% to 80% of your maximum heart rate.

Aerobic Exercise Basics

Fitness: Fitness is a general term which has different meanings for different people, depending on their sex, age, heredity, activity level and disease condition. Endurance is key to good fitness. For the fibromyalgia or chronic pain patient, fitness is defined simply as the ability to perform activities of daily living without feelings of exertion or fatigue.

Endurance: Endurance is defined as the ability to perform work for a prolonged period of time while resisting fatigue. Your body's level of oxygen utilization will determine your level of endurance. The amount of oxygen your body gets each minute ultimately depends on your cardiovascular fitness. Fitness of the cardiovascular sysem can be greatly enhanced by exercising at your target heart rate for a prolonged period of time.

Aerobic Exercise: This is the next step up from a moderate-intensity activity. Aerobic exercise is simply an extended activity that makes you breathe harder and your heart beat faster. The best aerobic exercise is any activity you enjoy and can perform for about 20 minutes at your target heart rate.

Examples include:

- Brisk walking
- Jogging
- Bicycling
- Stair climbing

- Aerobic dance
- Skiing

Target Heart Rate

Your *maximum* heart rate is determined by subtracting your age from 220. Your *target* heart rate is the rate you achieve through exercise within a range of 60% to 80% of your maximum heart rate. For example, if you are 40 years old, your maximum heart rate is 180 (220 − 40). You should exercise and aim for 108 to 144 beats per minute (60% to 80% of 180).

Target Heart Rate By Age

AGE	60%	80%
30	114	152
35	111	148
40	108	144
45	105	140
50	102	136
55	99	132
60	96	128
65	93	124

How to measure heart rate: Exercise for a while. Stop and place the first two fingers (not thumb) of one hand on the base of the thumb in front of the wrist of opposite hand. Locate a pulse. Watch the second indicator of your watch. Count your pulse for 15 seconds, then multiply this count by 4 to get your heart rate.

Types of Aerobics Programs

High-impact aerobics: Aerobics in which both feet come off the ground in different choreography styles.

Low-impact aerobics (recommended for fibromyalgia patients): Aerobic exercise in which one foot is always planted firmly on the ground.

Body-sculpting aerobics: Aerobic exercise combined with free weight exercise program, aimed at toning the body and improving muscular strength.

Funk aerobics: A combination of low- and high-impact dance movements. It can be rock, or cardio-funk.

Muscle-Strengthening Exercise (Progressive Resistance Exercise)

This is defined as any form of exercise or activity in which muscle action (whether static or dynamic) is opposed by an outside force. Muscles gain strength, endurance, and power when they habitually work against an opposite force like gravity, free weights, ankle weights, etc.

You need muscle-strengthening activity in order to develop endurance or fight fatigue during the performance of daily activities.

The term "muscle strengthening" usually conjures up images of weird-looking muscle builders and spending several hours at the gym every day. The fact of the matter is that you don't need anything more than mild strengthening to tone your body and build endurance. However, you need to be regular at it and maintain a consistent schedule.

Sample Muscle-strenthening Program

A. To strengthen the extensor group of muscles of the wrist, arms, neck, back and hips.

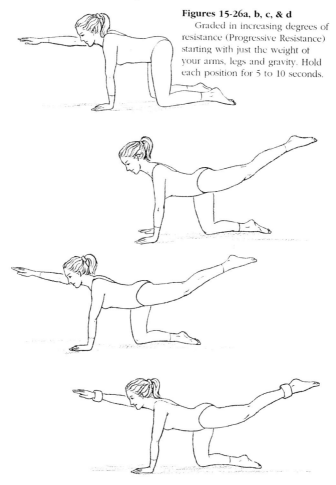

Figures 15-26a, b, c, & d
Graded in increasing degrees of resistance (Progressive Resistance) starting with just the weight of your arms, legs and gravity. Hold each position for 5 to 10 seconds.

B. *To strengthen the flexor group of muscles—(abdominal muscles, hip muscles, thighs).*

Figures 15-27a, b, & c.
Lie on the floor or a bed. Gradually increase resistance as shown.

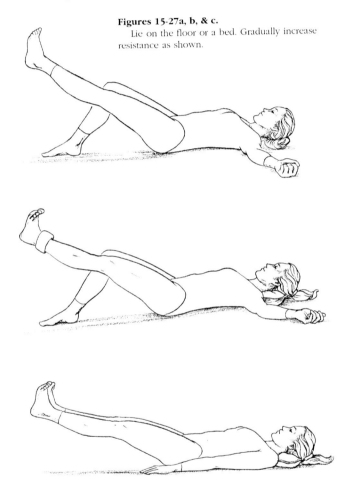

C. To isolate and strengthen large muscle groups of the limbs.

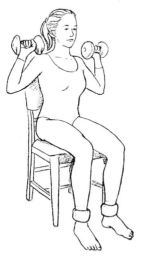

Figure 15-28
Use cuff weights strapped around your ankles and wrists or work out with dumbbells as shown.

A. Grasp a dumbbell in each hand as shown. Raise the dumbbells to shoulder height. From this starting position, raise the dumbbells above your head until your elbows are fully extended. Repeat 10 to 20 times (as tolerated.

B. Strap a lightweight weight cuff around each ankle. Raise legs alternately until knees are fully extended. Hold for 5 to 10 seconds. Repeat 10 times.

How to Benefit Fully from your Exercise and Fitness Program

Set Sensible Goals

Stay motivated by reminding yourself often about the benefits you hope to achieve if you persevere in your program. Actually write them down and read them often. Set sensible, achievable short-term goals, like being able to mop your kitchen floor without fatigue.

- Maintain an exercise journal. Write down symptoms and problems encountered. You may need to discuss these with your doctor, trainer or physical therapist.

- Reward yourself each time you are able to achieve a goal.

A good motivation for hanging in there is the thought of the immense relief you will get from depressive moods, pain, and fatigue, and improvement in your sleep quality. The list is endless. Most importantly, this is the only way I know by which you can completely take back your life from fibromyalgia.

Maintain a Fitness-Conscious Lifestyle

Here are some tips:

- Create situations that will make you exercise, like parking your car far away from your destination, so you get to walk a distance.

- Spend time with the kids outdoors if the weather permits.

- Find an exercise partner who is at the same fitness level as you are and take long walks together.

- Use the stairs instead of the elevator whenever you can.

- Include some form of exercise activity in your daily activity planner. A sample program can be:

  - 20 minutes of stretching and aerobics 3 times per week.

  - Strengthening and activity (walking) 2 times per week.

At the least, endeavor to include 20 minutes of aerobics two times a week. Stretching can be done any time you like.

CHAPTER 16

⁓

Fast Solutions for Muscle Soreness, Headaches and Sleep Problems

Solutions for Muscle Soreness

Get a Good Night's Sleep

Getting a good night's sleep may be the solution for most muscle soreness problems. In fibromyalgia, for example, muscle soreness can be traced to lack of restorative sleep. As discussed earlier in this book, the deep phase of sleep is required for the repairing hormone from the pituitary gland to become effective in repairing muscle micro-trauma. Therefore, forming a good sleep hygiene habit would go a long way in alleviating this problem.

Mind Your Posture

The postural muscles of your body are in constant tension, both static and dynamic, in maintaining your erect body in space against the pull of gravity. These muscles function optimally when your body is balanced over its center of gravity. In the balanced position, muscles in all areas of the body are in equilibrium and contract efficiently. For example, if you stoop when you walk and move beyond this line of gravity, muscles in the back must contract to prevent you from falling forward.

If poor posture becomes habitual, the opposing muscles sometimes become tired and sore. In order to relieve this fatigue and soreness, you must manage the predisposing factor, which is poor posture.

121

Good Posture Hints

- Watch your head position. Correct it and the rest of the body will follow. Gently tuck in your chin as you stretch the muscles at the back of the neck.

- Brace and pull your shoulders backward.

- Practice often at aligning your ear, shoulder, hip and ankle. Visualize an imaginary line that passes through these four structures; your task is to maintain it in a straight line.

- Always remember to sit straight, while maintaining the natural inward curve of your lower back. Also make sure your car's seat is ergonomically designed to assist you in maintaining a correct posture. If not, buy a posture correction insert.

- Sleep on a mattress that is firm enough not to sag under your weight, and soft enough to adapt to the natural curves of your body. If you suffer from back pain, you might consider sleeping in a "neutral" or "zero gravity" position (see figure 14-3 in Chapter 14).

- Change positions often; that is, don't stand or sit for more than 20 minutes at a time.

- *Shoes:* Avoid high-heeled shoes, platform shoes, high boots and shoes with inflexible soles.

- *Bags and weights:* Avoid heavy luggage; ask someone to help you. Don't strap bags over your shoulders. Keep them close to the body. If you have to lift, bend at the knees instead of the waist.

- *Bras:* Heavy breasts tend to pull a woman forward and promote a round-shouldered posture. Wear a strong bra that crosses over at the back. Don't let it fit too tightly around the chest or over the shoulders, because this can restrict blood flow or put pressure on spinal nerves.

Take Warm Baths

Soak yourself in a warm aromatic bath for about an hour. Set a timer in case you fall asleep and hurt yourself. You can also light an aromatic candle and listen to relaxation music.

Try Over-the-counter Medication

Try purchasing over-the-counter medicines first, before using addictive prescription painkillers. Be on a SAM-e supplementation program. Medical research has proven that SAM-e can relieve muscle pain even better than a TENS unit.

Use a TENS unit

This is a kind of electrical stimulator used in most physical therapy centers. You may have to order such a unit through a physical therapist or your physician.

Try Trigger Point Injections

An anti-inflammatory steroid can be injected directly into the painful site. I am not sure how helpful this can be for fibromyalgia pain, which is essentially different from inflammatory symptoms.

Perform Breathing/Muscle Relaxation Exercises

Breathing exercises have an overall calming effect on your system. More oxygen eventually gets to your muscles. Minor muscle spasms may have created muscle tension and pain. Twenty minutes of deep muscle relaxation exercise (see Chapter 14) can perform miracles on your pain.

Headaches

It is very important that you are thoroughly evaluated for the cause or causes of regular headaches. Find a physician who has some experience with headaches and has a headache program or clinic.

If you experience nausea, drowsiness, vomiting and fever along with your headaches, you really need to be evaluated by a doctor. Causes of headaches can range from mild spasms of the head and neck muscles to very serious disease conditions. Standard painkillers usually relieve regular headaches. There are also medications that resolve blood vessel changes, etc. Some self-help strategies include:

- Managing stress and muscle tension (see Chapter 14);
- Checking for allergies and sensitivity to particular substances or foods;
- Getting plenty of fresh air, enough sleep and rest;
- Avoiding caffeine and any other foods that have been known to trigger your headaches. Keep a headache diary in which you make note of foods you have eaten, events that have taken place, and activities you have performed preceding the onset of a headache;
- Checking your pillow and neck posture while sleeping. Get appropriate neck support or pillow;
- Getting a deep massage. You can also use a massager. Some come with a heat and vibration control;
- Using aromatherapy. Lavender essential oil mixed with almond oil can be used to massage head and neck muscles. Other oils commonly used include peppermint and eucalyptus;
- Performing breathing exercises. Chronic headaches result in fatiguing of head and neck muscles due to constant tension. This reduces muscle blood flow as blood vessels are contracted. Less oxygen gets to the muscles and lactic acid builds up. This causes more pain and tension as the vicious cycle continues. Deep diaphragmatic breathing and rest can break up this cycle.

Sleep Problems

Lack of sleep, otherwise called insomnia, is a common human problem that affects about 10% to 15% of the population, mostly women. There are several types of insomnia, including:

- Problem with initiating sleep;
- Problem with remaining asleep;
- Circadian rhythm problems;
- Restless legs and other uncontrollable muscle activity associated with sleep;
- And of course lack of the deep phase of sleep, leading to unrestorative sleep.

In order to accurately diagnose insomnia, a medical expert needs to conduct a thorough evaluation. It may be necessary to be tested in a sleep laboratory. Many prescription sleep medications are very addictive. Addiction can manifest itself in as little as one week of medication.

In minor cases of insomnia, the problem can be resolved with regular relaxation training and deep breathing exercises. Sleep, as a biological process, should not be controlled or made to happen; rather, it should be allowed to happen by observing some simple practices of good sleep hygiene:

- Avoid caffeine, alcohol, nicotine and other chemical stimulants.
- Don't watch television, especially intense programs, just before bedtime.
- Put a leash on your mind; avoid worrying during bedtime; limit your worrying to a designated "worry time."
- Get plenty of exercise or aerobic activity during the day. Don't exercise, however, too close to your bedtime. Finish exercising at least four hours before you turn in for the night.
- Take a walk in the early morning sunshine. This may help reset your body's internal clock.

- Practice prayer and meditation.
- Avoid prolonged naps during the day. This will impair quality of your sleep later in the day.
- Let the bedroom be a good place to sleep. Avoid turning it into something else, like another office. Improve on your bedroom environment with soft sleep aids, pillows and assistive devices that can assist you in relaxing.
- Create a pre-sleep program or ritual, such as reading a passage from a helpful book, listening to soft music, etc.
- Eat lightly before bedtime. Too much food close to your bedtime, is enough to prevent you from falling asleep.
- Endeavor to maintain a regular bedtime and waking time.
- Maintain a neutral or zero gravity sleeping posture. This will reduce muscle tension significantly.
- If you think you have sleep apnea, get medical assistance to correct the problem.
- Take a long, warm bath or steam bath before sleep time.
- I personally find relaxation sound tapes (waterfalls, rains, forest sounds) very helpful in achieving good sleep.

CHAPTER 17

~

Nutritional Healing

The quality of our lives is very much affected by what we eat or inhale, so much so that to a very large extent, what we know as "alternative medicine" has been built on the manipulation of what we eat and drink.

Our bodies require all sorts of nutrients to survive – for energy, growth and tissue repair. Our bodies are composed largely of water, which acts as a medium for blood and plasma, transporting nutrients into tissue cells and evacuating their waste products.

Macronutrients are comprised of protein, fats and carbohydrates. Proteins are required for tissue growth and maintenance and the formation of several hormones and enzymes. Fat, on the other hand, provides energy, insulates organs, and assists with the utilization of certain vitamins. Carbohydrates are the body's chief energy reservoir.

Micronutrients include vitamins and minerals. These nutrients, even though needed in small amounts, are vital to the body's health. Prolonged deficiency can cause numerous health problems.

Other Methylation Boosters Besides SAM-e

Many people complain about the exorbitant cost of SAM-e. In fact, regular supplementation with SAM-e can cost upward of $200 per month. As an alternative, it is important to note that other nutrients are quite capable of boosting methylation.

Folic Acid, Vitamin B6, (Pyridoxal S-phosphate)
and Vitamin B12 (Cobalamin)

These nutrients play a major role in assisting the body to achieve an optimal utilization of SAM-e. They also play a major role in the breakdown of a harmful amino acid called *homocysteine.*

Homocysteine can be beneficial in small amounts, since it is associated with transsulfuration and methylation reactions. The homocysteine molecule contains highly useful sulfur substrates. Excessive amounts, however, can lead to serious liver and heart problems.

Homocysteine levels in the body are controlled through enzymatic degradation. This process requires adequate levels of folate and vitamins B_6 and B_{12} to maintain a normal balance between homocysteine and SAM-e. Or, as you take SAM-e, you might want to includes a 'B' complex multivitamin.

According to recent medical research, you will need about 650 micrograms of folic acid daily in order to significantly lower homocysteine levels in your system. A British study, using a large number of participants, reported a dramatic reduction in their homocysteine levels with a dosage of 500 micrograms of folic acid.

How to Use B_6, B_{12} and Folic Acid

These are produced in different varieties and shapes, tablets and capsules, either singly or as B-complex preparations. An effective dosage is 500 to 750 micrograms of folic acid.

According to Ms. Corinne Netzer's *Big Book of Medical Cures,* it is better to take all three, since they cooperate and influence each other.

Are There Any Side Effects?

Of course, as they say, too much of a good thing is bad. Very high doses of the 'B' vitamins may cause gas, bloating, gastric upsets and diarrhea. Also, long-term usage can cause kidney problems. So check with your doctor if you are taking more than 800 micrograms of folic acid daily.

Fibromyalgia Symptoms and Supplements to Alleviate Them

Many alternative health practitioners believe strongly that the key to fibromyalgia care is well-planned nutrition and supplementation. Besides SAM-e, several other nutrients have been found helpful for the following fibromyalgia symptoms:

- Muscle soreness;
- Sleep problems;
- Chronic fatigue;
- Cognitive impairment, also called fibro-fog;
- Headaches and migraines;
- Irritable bowel syndrome.

Muscle Soreness

Several theories have been postulated about the cause of muscle soreness in fibromyalgia. Most of them point to a lack of restorative sleep as the culprit. Muscle soreness is normally remedied during the deep phase of sleep, also known as Stage 4, by the action of a hormone secreted by the pituitary gland. Another theory implicates a local lack of oxygen by muscle tissues, leading to a decrease of glycogen breakdown and the synthesis of ATP. Because of the aforementioned theories, many experts believe adequate supplementation with malic acid and magnesium would resolve muscle pain or soreness.

Malic Acid

We normally get *malic acid* into our bodies through our diets. It can also be produced in small quantities by our bodies during the citric acid cycle. Malic acid is very important for energy production during both aerobic and anaerobic processes. Actually, a research study was undertaken to determine its effects under diminished muscle oxygen states (as in fibromyalgia). The researchers noticed significant improvement within 48 hours at a dosage of 1200 to 2400 mg of malic acid.

How to take malic acid: It comes in tablets of 250 mg each. Take 500 to 750 mg of malic acid about 1 hour before breakfast and another 500 mg before dinner.

Magnesium

Magnesium is the most important supplement for energy production and mitochondria health. Low levels of magnesium can disrupt ATP production. Because ATP energizes the movement of magnesium into cells, a vicious cycle is set in motion which further hampers ATP synthesis. Several studies seem to suggest that magnesium, when combined with malic acid, reduced tender points by 41% after only four weeks of treatment.

How to take magnesium: Magnesium comes in tablet form. It may be combined with other nutrients as a multivitamin. An effective daily dose is about 300 to 600 mg, usually taken with regular meals to encourage optimal absorption.

Side effects: May cause stomach upsets and diarrhea.

Sleep Problems

As discussed already, non-restorative sleep is a primary cause of the symptoms of fibromyalgia. This type of sleep deprivation is characterized by the situation in which the deep phase of sleep is interrupted by awake-like bursts of brain activity. Recommended supplements include melatonin and valerian root.

Melatonin

Melatonin is produced naturally by the pineal gland. Besides being a powerful anti-oxidant, it greatly affects the body's sleep/awake cycle. It has been found to be a good sleep problem remedy without the side effects associated with sleeping pills.

How to take melatonin: It comes in tablet form of 2.5 mg each, usually as a small sublingual tablet. Take one tablet at bedtime.

Boosting your melatonin level naturally: Melatonin has a Dracula-like attitude: Its level rises with the sunset and continues through the night. Then it starts to decrease with daylight. This, in turn, triggers neural impulses, which slow melatonin production.

Besides this rhythmic cycle of light and darkness, other factors, like daily routine, may play some role. Some experts suggest the following lifestyle habits may boost melatonin's natural production:

- Eat meals regularly. This will ensure a regular body rhythm.

- Eat light meals at night. The digestion process slows down with melatonin production.

- Avoid stimulants like coffee, tea or caffeine-containing medicines.

- Don't exercise too late at night, as this can delay melatonin production. Take a walk outside at sunrise.

Caution with melatonin: Please be advised that melatonin is a powerful hormone. Any artificial regulation may have profound effects in your body. Dr. Gary Richardson, an assistant professor of medicine at Brown University, believes that supplementation of melatonin can add to your sleep problem. Melatonin falls within an FDA non-regulated area, and so certain dosages may increase the melatonin process to abnormal levels.

Valerian Root

Valerian root is known to have been used by ancient Greeks to cure insomnia. The Europeans use it for anxiety and restlessness, both of which can affect sleep quality.

Valerian root is derived from dried rhizomes and plant roots. It contains two distinct substances which affect the central nervous system—*vale potriates* and *sesquiterpenes*. They work by slowing down and sedating the central nervous system and the mind.

How to take valerian root: It comes in capsule form of 500 mg valerian root powder per capsule. Take 1 to 3 capsules (about 500-1500 mg), preferably with some food. Valerian root also comes as extracts, tinctures, or in teas.

Side effects: None. This makes valerian root a better sleep aid than melatonin.

Chronic Fatigue

Recommended supplements for chronic fatigue include NADH, CoEnzyme Q_{10}, malic acid, magnesium and L-carnitine.

NADH (Nicotinamide Adenine Dinucleotide)

Also known as CoEnzyme 1, this is a nutrient that is contained in our diet. It is a nutrient that can enhance the production of dopamine and some other transmitters, and also assist in the cells' process of converting food to energy. Dr. Jorg Birkmayer, director of the Birkmayer Institute for Parkinson's Therapy in Vienna, has been using NADH to treat patients with chronic fatigue syndrome, among other ailments. He usually prescribes 10 mg of NADH daily before breakfast and has reported significant improvements in patient health within 8 to 12 weeks of treatment.

Another clinician, Dr. Joseph Bellanti of Georgetown University Immunology Center in Washington, DC, found good results in a study involving 26 patients with chronic fatigue syndrome. Nineteen of those studied reported significant improvements in their conditions

Recommended dosage: Take 5 to 10 mg. It usually comes in tablet form. There are no known adverse effects or contra-indications.

CoEnzyme Q_{10}

This nutrient is produced naturally in the body, and stored in concentrated amounts within the heart muscles. CoEnzyme

Q_{10} is also found in foods, especially organ meats. It is an important nutrient for the body's energy conversion processes like ATP synthesis. It also aids electron transport processes across the mitochondria. Another CoEnzyme Q_{10} function is to act as a powerful antioxidant within the body.

It is particularly beneficial for heart conditions. It bolsters the heart. It does this by increasing the heart's energy output, making it stronger. Dr. William Lee called it "the ultimate antidote to aging." Some researchers also believe it may play a role in breast cancer recurrence prevention. CoEnzyme Q_{10} also assists in boosting the body's immune response system.

How to take CoEnzyme Q_{10}: It is usually packaged in softgels of 100 mg each or capsules of 30 to 50 mg each. Cardiologists usually recommend a dosage of 100 to 300 mg of CoEnzyme Q_{10} daily for heart patients. About 100 mg (one softgel) is recommended for chronic fatigue syndrome and fibromyalgia sufferers. Regular supplementation of CoEnzyme Q_{10} for the healthy should be about 30 to 60 mg daily.

L-Carnitine

This is produced in the liver and kidneys. Its function within the body includes fatty acid transfer into cells for energy production. Therefore, regular supplementation with L-carnitine would enhance the processes of fat transport and metabolism. Dr. Plioplys reported significant improvements in 12 out of 18 chronic fatigue patients he treated with L-carnitine.

This nutrient is known to lower cholesterol levels in the blood; boost the body against stress; and support kidney, heart and liver functions. It also promotes the body's ability to endure prolonged physical activity.

How to take L-Carnitine: Packaged in 250 mg capsules. Take 1 to 3 capsules daily.

Cognitive Impairment (Fibro-fog)

Cognitive impairment, also called "fibro-fog" among fibromyalgia syndrome sufferers, is a term that describes a gradual short-term memory loss. Patients begin to forget simple things like where they parked their cars or the fact that they have appointments.

A brain deprived of adequate amounts of oxygen, glucose and other nutrients malfunctions, just like any other organ. Its information processing system becomes impaired.

Probable causes of this in fibromyalgia patients include:

- Insufficient blood supply to the brain;
- Stress, which produces excessive amounts of cortisol, which in turn interferes with memory;
- Poor nutritional habits;
- Medications being used.

Probable nutritional remedies include ginkgo biloba, phosphatidyl choline, and acetyl L-carnitine.

Ginkgo Biloba

Ginkgo is known to be the oldest living tree species found on Earth. This tree is believed to contain several antioxidants, like flavonoids such as rutin and quercetin, which assist in the degradation of free radicals.

Flavonoids also improve brain blood flow by strengthening capillaries. They prevent the accumulation of brain fluids and activate the brain's chemical messengers.

An ancient Chinese and European remedy was scientifically tested in a major study by LeBars and associates at the New York Institute of Medical Research. About 309 patients with severe memory problems following stroke and Alzheimer's were tested in the study. After one year of observation, the researchers reported significant improvements in many subjects from the patient group in areas of memory, reasoning, and social functioning over members of the placebo group. They also observed that supplementation with ginkgo biloba was able to arrest the progress of cognitive impairment in some subjects.

How to take ginkgo biloba: Ginkgo biloba is packaged in different forms. The best is capsule form. Take 120 mg daily for memory problems. No side effects have been reported.

Phosphatidyl Choline

This is a major substrate of lecithin. It promotes the emulsification and degradation of fat deposits. Due to this function, phosphatidyl choline is helpful in preventing heart problems—the narrowing of arteries. It also assists in the prevention of liver diseases and gall stones. According to clinical studies, memory impairment can be improved with a 3 g daily dose.

How to take phosphatidyl choline: This supplement is packaged in softgels of 420 mg each. Take about 420 to 840 mg daily (that is, one to two softgels). Pregnant patients should check with their obstetricians, since it may be contraindicated during pregnancy.

Acetyl L-Carnitine

This is another naturally occurring substance. Although related to carnitine, it has a different chemical composition. It is another antioxidant and assists in degradation of free radicals. Other functions include promotion of cell health by assisting in cellular energy production.

Dr. Jay Pattegrew of the University of Pittsburgh School of Medicine conducted a clinical study in which 3000 mg of acetyl L-carnitine was used to treat several patients with some form of cognitive impairment for one year. He compared the results from this group against that of the placebo group. He found that the acetyl L-carnitine group performed better on a battery of cognitive status tests than the placebo group. This led Dr. Pattegrew and associates to believe that acetyl L-carnitine may be able to halt memory loss progress in Alzheimer's patients.

How to take acetyl L-Carnitine: Acetyl L-carnitine is usually packaged in capsules. There are no government dosage guidelines. Clinicians recommend a dosage of 1000 to 3000 mg daily. For best results, take in divided doses throughout the day, on an empty stomach.

Side effects: No known serious ones. Very few people have reported nausea and vomiting.

Headaches and Migraines

Causes of headaches and migraines are several and varied. A thorough medical examination by a headache expert and physician is required. This is because the headaches and migraines may be symptoms of a more severe health problem. Also, a comprehensive evaluation is a pre-condition for an effective headache remedy.

Migraine headache: Pain is caused by changes in blood vessels of the temples. This pain can last for days. Symptoms besides headache include visual problems, nausea and dizziness.

Cluster headache: This is similar to a migraine and is also caused by blood vessel changes. Pain is intense and localized around one eye. Pain is intermittent; that is, it goes and comes back after a few hours. It is known to last for a long time. Nobody is sure what causes it.

Tension headache: This type of headache is usually caused by stress and muscle tension, especially tension in the muscles of head and neck. It can also have other causes, like exposure to environmental toxins.

Nutritional remedies for headaches include feverfew and magnesium.

Feverfew

This nutrient has over a two-thousand-year history among herbalists of different cultures. Ancient Greeks used it for painful menstrual periods. It has been used since the 1970s in America and Canada in the prevention or relief of painful headaches. It is especially effective for migraine headaches, but can also affect blood vessels and consequently relieve other headache symptoms.

The first known scientific study that proved the effectiveness of feverfew on migraine was conducted by Johnson and associates in 1985 and reported in the *British Medical Journal*. Seventeen migraine sufferers who had been on a diet of feverfew leaves (which they chewed) were divided into two groups. One group received feverfew capsules (instead of leaves); the other group received a placebo. On reevaluation after a time, results showed no change in the feverfew group, while the placebo group got worse. Due to this result, the researchers concluded that feverfew was beneficial for headache relief, and it didn't matter whether one took it in capsule form or chewed leaves instead.

How to take feverfew: It is packaged in capsule or tablet forms. It can also be chewed as dried or fresh leaves. There may be some irritation of the mouth for some.

Dosage: Purchase a standardized brand, usually standardized with 0.2% of parthenolide as an active ingredient. Take a daily dose of 250 micrograms of parthenolide or check manufacturer's dosage specification.

Adverse effects: You may be allergic to it. It may cause rashes or some itching in some people. Pregnant women should be careful and might be better off discussing it with their obstetricians, since feverfew can cause uterine contractions.

Magnesium

Research findings indicate some headache sufferers have low levels of magnesium in their systems and supplementation with it has been observed to bring relief from headaches. Mauskop and fellow investigators gave 1000 mg of magnesium intravenously to a group of 40 headache patients which included children, women and men. The results indicated that headache symptoms were completely eliminated in about 80% of participants in the study. Already, magnesium is known to relieve symptoms like hypersensitivity to light and nausea.

How to take magnesium for headaches: Magnesium comes in tablet form. It can also be combined with other nutrients as a multivitamin preparation. Optimal dosage, according to several studies, is 360 to 600 mg daily, taken at meal time.

Adverse effects: Usually safe. May cause stomach irritation and diarrhea. Magnesium is contraindicated for people with heart and kidney problems.

Irritable Bowel Syndrome

Formerly known as spastic colon or mucous colitis. Symptoms include cramps, bloating, gas and changes in bowel habits. Some IBS patients have constipation or diarrhea or both. The medical textbooks say there is no cure. I say perhaps there is, only one hasn't been found yet. Some have also called it a functional disorder and not really a disease, since the colon shows no sign of a disease on examination. But whatever the medical community chooses to call it, I would not trivialize the serious problems sufferers face continually.

Nutritional Remedies

A proper and well-planned diet may relieve symptoms. If you are a sufferer, it is a good idea to maintain a journal of what helps it get better and the things that make it worse, and discuss these dietary components with your physician. A dietician can be consulted to assist you in planning an adequate diet, but do not sacrifice your normal nutritional balance just because you are worried about IBS symptoms. That is, don't "cut off your nose to spite your face." Dietary fiber may help. Whole grain breads, cereals, fruits, beans and vegetables are excellent sources of fiber.

High-fiber diets relieve IBS by mildly distending the colon, thereby preventing intestinal spasms from developing. Fiber also can retain water in stools, thereby making them easier to evacuate.

Peppermint Oil

This substance contains a large quantity of menthol, which is an ancient remedy for intestinal problems. Menthol appears to slow down cramping muscle spasms and also relieves indigestion and diarrhea.

How to take peppermint oil: It is packaged in gelatin or coated capsules. Gelatin packaging is preferred since it will disintegrate easily once in the stomach environment.

For IBS take an enteric-coated capsule. This will allow it to bypass the stomach and break up within the colon, where its action is needed.

For dosage guidelines, please observe the manufacturer's specifications.

Adverse effects: There are no known adverse effects.

Psyllium

Also called plantago and ispaghula. Psyllium is primarily used as a laxative and to treat diarrhea. One study, involving 26 IBS patients, reported some relief of irritable bowel syndrome symptoms in about 20 of the participants in the study.

Dosage: Follow manufacturer's guidelines.

Good Health Starts with a Good Diet

The Food Guide Pyramid

The main objective of diet plans is to achieve and maintain an adequate body composition, which will provide an adequate capacity for physical and mental work. The daily requirement of essential nutrients depends on several variables, like sex, age, height, weight, metabolic and activity levels.

In order to determine an adequate nutritional variation for Americans, the Food and Nutrition Board of the National Academy of Sciences—National Research Council and the US Department of Agriculture analyzed information and data on 45 essential nutrients in people on special diets and came up with the following Food Guide Pyramid.

The Food Guide Pyramid

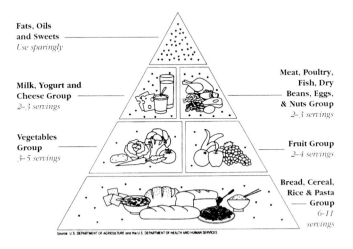

Fats, Oils and Sweets
Use sparingly

Milk, Yogurt and Cheese Group
2–3 servings

Vegetables Group
3–5 servings

Meat, Poultry, Fish, Dry Beans, Eggs, & Nuts Group
2–3 servings

Fruit Group
2–4 servings

Bread, Cereal, Rice & Pasta Group
6-11 servings

Source: U.S. DEPARTMENT OF AGRICULTURE and the U.S. DEPARTMENT OF HEALTH AND HUMAN SERVICES

What Counts as a Serving?*

Grain Products Group
(bread, cereal, rice, and pasta)

- One slice of bread
- 1 ounce of ready-to-eat cereal
- ½ cup of cooked cereal, rice, or pasta

---

* Some foods fit into more than one group. Dried beans, peas, and lentils can be counted as servings in either the meat and beans group or the vegetable group. These "crossover" foods can be counted as servings from either one or the other group, but not both. Serving sizes indicated here are those used in the Food Guide Pyramid and based on both suggested and usually consumed portions necessary to achieve adequate nutrient intake. They differ from serving sizes on the Nutrition Facts Label, which reflect the size of portions usually consumed.

Vegetable Group

- 1 cup of raw leafy vegetables
- ½ cup of other vegetables—cooked or chopped raw
- ½ cup of vegetable juice

Fruit Group

- 1 medium apple, banana, orange
- ½ cup of chopped, cooked, or canned fruit
- ½ cup of fruit juice

Milk Group
(milk, yogurt, and cheese)

- 1 cup of milk or yogurt
- 1½ ounces of natural cheese
- 2 ounces of processed cheese

Meat and Beans Group
(meat, poultry, fish, dry beans, eggs, and nuts)

- 2-3 ounces of cooked lean meat, poultry, or fish
- ½ cup of cooked dried beans or 1 egg counts as 1 ounce of lean meat. Two tablespoons of peanut butter or ⅓ cup of nuts count as 1 ounce of meat.

In summary, the pyramid offers the following advice to Americans:

- Choose a diet with plenty of grain products, vegetables and fruits.
- Choose a diet that is low in fat, saturated fat and cholesterol.
- Eat a variety of foods.
- Choose a diet that is moderate in salt and sodium.
- Choose a diet that is moderate in sugars.
- If you drink alcoholic beverages, please do so in moderation.

Above all, balance what you consume with adequate physical activity, or else you will be climbing a mountain you'll have a tough time coming down from. Realistically, there are no safe fixes or medications that can make the fat "go away." If you put it on, be prepared to take it off with exercise and the safe correction of poor nutritional habits.

PART 5

Fibromyalgia
Disability Issues
and
Conclusions

CHAPTER 18

~

Fibromyalgia Disability Issues: How to File Claims Successfully

The Social Security Administration (SSA) routinely denies fibromyalgia disability claims. One major reason for this is that fibromyalgia sufferers have a hard time proving that they are disabled in accordance with SSA criteria. Other reasons include:

- Lack of current work capacity documentation in medical records;
- Lack of objective and quantifiable laboratory findings;
- Constant fatigue and poor endurance are not considered strong enough disability indicators;
- Many physicians fail to document clear evidence of disability.

The Social Security Administration is known to routinely deny fibromyalgia-related disability claims applications except where there are other disabling diagnoses with supporting laboratory data. However, this is not the case in countries like Canada and many European countries, where fibromyalgia is regarded as a disabling condition.

Therefore, in order to file claims successfully you, your lawyer and physician must function as a team in providing needed medical information, especially evidence of *total disability*. This means you cannot function in a recent job and cannot be retrained for any equivalent alternative jobs. The physician's notes are crucial to a successful outcome, but unfortunately, many patients change doctors midstream. Most sufferers understandably differ in opinion as to their healthcare strategies and priorities. And so, there may be cases of patients' non-compliance to their doctors' prescriptions, etc.

Available research data seem to suggest that about 30% of fibromyalgia sufferers change jobs because of their condition. Seventeen percent of them can no longer perform in their previous jobs. A research study by Wolfe and associates indicates that about 26% of fibromyalgia patients reported receiving one form of disability payment or another. This number increased to 46.4% after 1988. A closer look at this national trend revealed that the San Antonio and Los Angeles areas had the highest records of approved disability claims applications.

The Fibromyalgia Impact Questionnaire (FIQ)

A very good solution to the perennial problem of lack of disability documentation in fibromyalgia disability insurance claims is the Fibromyalgia Impact Questionnaire (FIQ). (See table 18-1.) The FIQ, in its original form, is a 10-item self-administered questionnaire that can objectively document depression, functional capacity, work capacity, anxiety, sleep, pain, stiffness, fatigue and general well-being. In fact, the FIQ is actually an adaptation from a commonly used arthritis impact questionnaire.

The FIQ is considered an effective tool for the following reasons:

- It is very practical and takes only a short time to complete.
- Its comprehensive nature takes fibromyalgia's multisymptomatic nature into consideration.
- Researchers have proven the FIQ to be valid and reliable (that is, it is able to measure what it is supposed to measure).

How to Use the FIQ

As a fibromyalgia sufferer, you and your treatment team can use the FIQ to:

- Monitor your fibromyalgia progress.
- Document progress in measurable, quantifiable terms. This is a crucial factor in the success of your receipt of payment from insurance companies. These companies habitually deny claims for chronic pain cases.

Table 18-1: Fibromyalgia Impact Questionnaire
(Modified from *Journal of Rheumatology*. (1991). 18, 728-733.)

Name: _____

Date: _____

Instructions: For questions 1 through 10, please check the number that best describes how you did overall for the past week. If you don't normally do something that is asked, check N/A.

1. **Were you able to:**

	Most Always	Times	Occasi- onally	Never	Not Applicable
a. Go shopping?	0	1	2	3	N/A
b. Do laundry with a washer and dryer?	0	1	2	3	N/A
c. Prepare meals?	0	1	2	3	N/A
d. Wash dishes/ cooking utensils by hand?	0	1	2	3	N/A
e. Vacuum a rug?	0	1	2	3	N/A
f. Make beds?	0	1	2	3	N/A
g. Walk several blocks?	0	1	2	3	N/A
h. Visit friends and relatives?	0	1	2	3	N/A
i. Do yard work?	0	1	2	3	N/A
j. Drive a car?	0	1	2	3	N/A

2. **Of the days in the past week, how many days did you feel good?** (circle one)

    0   1   2   3   4   5   6   7

3. **How many days last week did you miss work because of your fibromyalgia?** (If you don't have a job outside the home, check N/A.)

    0   1   2   3   4   5   N/A

Instructions: For the following items, place a mark like this | at the point on the line that best indicates how you felt for the past week. Or you can also use numbers, like a scale of 1 to 10, 10 being the high end, or greatest amount, on the scale.

4. **When you did go to work, how much did pain or other symptoms of your fibromyalgia interfere with your ability to do your job?**

    No problem   Great difficulty
    with work   with work

5. **How bad has your pain been?**

    No pain   Very severe pain

6. **How tired have you been?**

    Not tired at all   Very tired

7. **How have you felt when you get up in the morning?**

    Awoke   Awoke
    well rested   very tired

8. **How bad has your stiffness been?**

    No stiffness   Very stiff

9. How nervous or anxious have you felt?

Not tense   Very tense

10. How depressed or blue have you felt?

Not depressed   Very depressed

11. Please indicate if you are taking any of the following for fibromyalgia:
    ☐ Tricyclics   ☐ Anti-inflammatory medications
    ☐ Other central nervous system medications
    ☐ Analgesics
    ☐ SAM-e or any other nutritional product

The Social Security Administration (SSA) and the Disability Insurance Program

---

Table 18-2: Social Security Administration Criteria for Disability Determination

The claimant must be unable to "engage in any substantial gainful activity* by reason of a medically determinable physical or medical impairment which can be expected to result in death or can be expected to last for a continuous period of at least 12 months."

The patient must have an impairment: "a demonstrable anatomy loss or abnormality of psychologic, physiologic or anatomic structures or function."

The impairment must be "demonstrable by medically acceptable clinical and laboratory diagnostic techniques. Symptoms alone cannot define an impairment."

From Social Security Regulations, 1986.

*"Substantial gainful activity" is regarded as working on a job on a regular payroll of at least $700/month.

Frequently Asked Questions and Answers About Disability Insurance:

Q: What are "SSDI" and "SSI"? Are they similar?
A: "SSDI" is an abbreviation for "Social Security Disability Insurance," while "SSI" stands for "Supplemental Security Income." The SSDI is a disability insurance program sponsored by the Social Security Administration (SSA) for workers who had worked for at least 5 years of the 10 years before becoming disabled. The program is funded by the "FICA" tax withheld from your paycheck.

The SSI is similar to SSDI and the SSA uses similar pre-qualification guidelines in determining acceptability. The only difference between the two is the financial requirement imposed in the SSDI.

Furthermore, the benefit amount paid by the SSDI is influenced by your length of employment and salary level, whereas the SSI sets only a certain fixed amount paid out before government-required deductions.

Some states may have other programs in place to supplement the SSDI.

Q: Does "other" or "supplementary" income affect the amount of disability income you receive?
A: According to Social Security Administration as well as disability attorney Scott Davis, it shouldn't, since the amount for which you qualify is based solely on your income in your previous job. That is, investment income, for example, doesn't count and does not affect the amount for which you qualify. Also, your spouse's income will not affect your SSDI benefits. However, spousal and other income *will* affect your SSI benefits, since this is a welfare program.

Q: How are SSDI, state disability insurance, Workers Compensation and private insurance programs related?
A. According to attorney Scott Davis, the following states offer programs for illnesses and disabilities not caused by work: New

Jersey, New York, Rhode Island, Hawaii, California and Puerto Rico. These states provide assistance before the SSDI program kicks in. Amounts paid are usually small and limited in duration, for example, 26 weeks in New Jersey and Hawaii. Please call your state's appropriate agency for further details.

Workers Compensation programs require that your illness be work-related, which the SSDI does not require. However, the SSDI does require that you have been unable to work for at least 12 months. Workers Compensation can pay for partial disability, but the SSDI requires you to be totally disabled before you can become eligible.

Private Disability Insurance: This is often provided by your employer, or, if not, you can fund it privately. Payment arrangements depend on the agreement in your policy. They may start disbursing benefits before any government programs. Amounts paid by private disability insurance may or may not be affected by the SSA benefits you receive.

Q: How do I know which type to apply for?
A: The Social Security Administration automatically determines the program for which it feels you are qualified.

Q: Can I continue to receive SSDI benefits after I reach retirement age, at 65?
A: The SSDI benefits cease when you reach 65 years. At this time, your retirement and Medicare payments take over.

Q: What happens if I have been self-employed? Will I be eligible for any benefits?
A: Yes, if you have paid your FICA and self-employment taxes, although it is common for many self-employed persons to neglect to do this.

Q: How large can these government benefits get?
A: As large as $240,000 by age 65, if you started receiving $1,000 monthly benefits at age 45 (according to attorney Scott Davis).

Application Package Requirements

According to another legal expert on this issue, Mr. W. J. Potter, in order to ensure a successful outcome to the application process, all concerned parties (claimant, her physician and attorney) must work as a team. There should be a singleness of purpose–that is, you must be prepared to go all the way. According to him, the system seems set up to poke holes in your application. Therefore, complete and detailed documentation of relevant information is crucial. In other words, your application package must contain the following information:

- Medical diagnosis;
- Past medical history;
- Types of medications taken or being taken;
- Present functional status;
- The history, nature and severity of pain;
- Past work history and current work capacity;
- Family status and current financial situation;
- Housing arrangement;
- Recreational lifestyle before and after fibromyalgia;
- How have you been coping with the problem.

The SSA focused medical review is aimed at finding out if there is about 90% reduction in your ability to perform at a job. Additionally, for you to be eligible for benefit payments, there should be sufficient evidence that your illness is chronic in nature. Your documentation should also include:

- Poor concentration at work;
- Memory impairments;
- Chronic disabling fatigue, etc.

It will be in your best interest if your doctor is aware of all the documentation needed right from the start.

Ineligibility Criteria

You will be considered ineligible for the disability insurance program under the following conditions:

- If you remain employed, even partially, in spite of fibromyalgia;
- If you were able to recover within 12 months of being diagnosed with fibromyalgia;
- If you have no definite medical diagnosis.

When Is the Best Time to File?

If it looks as if you won't be able to return to your job in 12 months, then file by the sixth month. The process is usually long and drawn out.

Disability Claim Application Process

STEP 1: Initial Application: If you were previously employed, and paid taxes, apply under Title II. If not, apply under Title XVI. Forward the application to your local Social Security district office either in person or by calling 800-772-1213.

Once your application is received and reviewed, the Social Security Administration will start gathering needed evidence.

STEP 2: Request for Reconsideration: If the initial application is denied (it would be wise to expect this), file a *request for reconsideration* within 60 days. You must note the jurisdictional nature of the timing. It means they will throw out your application if you can't beat the 60-day dateline. Send this application via your *disability claims attorney* to the Social Security Administration office. The SSA determines the maximum amount your lawyer can charge you for his services. Usually, attorneys get 25% of back benefits (from your illness onset) up to a maximum of $4,000. Miscellaneous charges (obtaining expert opinions, etc.) are not included.

STEP 3: Independent Examiner Evaluation: The SSA will then send you to be evaluated by its own experts, usually in contract

153

with the SSA. You may be denied again based on the expert's findings. The SSA will then suggest alternative employment.

STEP 4: Request for Hearing: After your *request for reconsideration* is denied, you will have 60 days (jurisdictional) to apply. Your case will then be forwarded to an *Administrative Judge,* who sets a trial date in about 4 months. That is, 4 months after your case file has been on his table, he sets a date for the hearing.

STEP 5: Trial: The trial is an evidentiary process in which you are allowed to provide both written documentation and oral presentation. Your physician's notes are examined. If this judge also denies your application, having determined you are not disabled within the law's criteria, you will again be able to appeal his decision within 60 days.

STEP 6: Appeals: Your case goes before the appeals council, which can give its verdict within 7 months. If you lose (that is, it affirms the trial judge's judgment), you will have the right to file suit.

STEP 7: Filing of Suit: You can file a suit after your appeal has been denied by the appeals council at the *United States District Court.* You must be represented by a properly licensed attorney; that is, licensed to practice at the US District Court. This Court may judge in your favor, and reverse the Administrative Judge's ruling, or may return your case for a new hearing, referred to as a *remand.* This process involves an examination of all the evidence submitted with the initial application at the district office.

Making Sure You Will Succeed

A very good way to make sure you will succeed is to make sure your physician writes detailed and complete notes. Your disability attorney will coordinate the efforts of all concerned in writing an appropriate narrative report.

Recently, the news has been good regarding successful applications and claims payment awards. A recent news release by the offices of Seattle-based Steven Krafchick, Esq., on November 30, 1999, announced a court victory on behalf of a disabled woman. This woman's disability payments had been cut off by her insurance company (Paul Revere). The woman, a 52-year-old former executive secretary, was diagnosed with fibromyalgia and chronic fatigue. Her policy promised her benefits if she became disabled up to 65 years of age. However, if she was diagnosed also with "psychiatric disorders," benefits would then be limited to only two years. So after some time of paying benefits, the Paul Revere insurance company sent her to their own experts, who promptly, as if on cue, labeled her a "psychiatric case."

The judge, Robert Lasnik, of the Federal Court in Seattle, gave judgment in her favor. According to the judge, the so-called expert, a neuro-psychologist, was not an MD, and did not consult the patient's physician. Neither did he review her complete medical history. And so, this expert could not have been able to determine her functional and psychological status or her work capacity. Paul Revere was then ordered to reinstate her benefits and pay her all accrued back benefits.

CHAPTER 19

~

Summary, Conclusions and Frequently Asked Questions about SAM-e and Fibromyalgia

Summary

I hope I have been successful in separating fact from fiction—and hype—about SAM-e and its role in the relief of fibromyalgia symptoms. The theme of this book has been that fibromyalgia syndrome is a multisymptomatic problem that requires an equally multifaceted treatment approach. SAM-e and the self-care non-drug strategies amply fit into this treatment model. It is my contention that in most cases, *addictive medications for a chronic and poorly understood health problem like fibromyalgia create more problems than they solve.* Furthermore, *there is no quick-fix single remedy for fibromyalgia;* rather, an effective medical treatment model must include:

- necessary lifestyle changes by the patient;
- patient empowerment self-care strategies, and
- a multidisciplinary cooperation.

To recap the important issues we have discussed:

- Pain can be helpful in prodding us to finally make health-enhancing lifestyle changes that we may have been putting off.
- Fibromyalgia is characterized by and differentiated from similar conditions by the fact that the pain it causes is generalized in more than one extremity, and the presence of so-called tender points.

- About 80% of all fibromyalgia sufferers are women between the ages of 25 and 55.

- There is no conclusive evidence on what causes fibromyalgia, and scientists are not certain that it is hereditary. Children can also suffer from a type called juvenile fibromyalgia.

- Conventional pharmacological remedies are known to cause substantial side effects, often precipitating withdrawal reactions and ultimately may cause more harm than good.

- SAM-e offers a safe alternative that is as effective as conventional pharmacological remedies, but without the unpleasant side effects.

- Pain is a constant complaint of fibromyalgia patients who would like to exercise. But exercise is mandatory to improving the quality of your life. This book has offered a safe and effective exercise and fitness guide that, of course, depends on your motivation, determination and perseverance.

- Nutrition is a very important aspect of fibromyalgia treatment. Many of the symptoms can be remedied by a well-planned diet and nutrition. The following supplements are particularly effective for fibromyalgia healing: folic acid, Vitamin B complex, malic acid, magnesium, valerian root, NADH, CoEnzyme Q_{10}, L-carnitine, ginko biloba, phosphatidyl choline, acetyl L-carnitine, feverfew, peppermint oil and psyllium.

Conclusions

Can fibromyalgia be cured? The standard textbook response is a negative. But I think this is wrong. It is not useful for our patients. It removes hope. The truth of the matter is that we don't know enough about fibromyalgia—what causes it or how it progresses—to pass such a definitive judgment. More research studies are needed. Also, there is still some controversy (especially between rheumatologists and neurologists) over whether the term "fibromyalgia syndrome" is a true diagnostic term at all. But having a diagnosis that differentiates it from similar or more serious conditions can offer some reassurance to patients.

Until a definite cure is found, SAM-e offers a lot of hope to the six million Americans who suffer from fibromyalgia. SAM-e, as we have shown, is involved in several metabolic processes that are fundamental to the body's natural self-healing systems.

Some Frequently Asked Questions about SAM-e and Fibromyalgia

Q: Can SAM-e cure fibromyalgia?
A: SAM-e alone cannot cure fibromyalgia. A multisymptomatic problem like FMS requires a multifaceted treatment method. SAM-e offers a safe alternative to conventional medications that are known to have unpleasant side effects and withdrawal reactions.

Q: How does SAM-e relieve fibromyalgia symptoms?
A: SAM-e may relieve fibromyalgia symptoms by indirectly influencing (through methylation and other metabolic processes) the factors that probably cause and maintain the condition of fibromyalgia.

Q: How can we supplement SAM-e through diet?
A: We don't actually supplement SAM-e in our diet due to the following reasons:

1. "Active methionine" is very limited in living organisms. SAM-e gets quickly used up once it gives away its methyl group.

2. SAM-e is highly unstable, and easily breaks down when we store or process our foods. Besides, too much ingestion of protein can cause the production of harmful metabolites like ammonia. Rather, we can enhance the process of methylation by consuming a proper diet. This

can be achieved by eating a well-balanced diet of soybeans, seeds, lentils, eggs, and protein-rich foods like fish and meat products. You must also take adequate amounts of other supplements like Vitamin B_{12}, B_6, folic acid and TMG (trimethyl-glycine).

Q: When can somebody have low levels of methylation?
A: Methylation is known to decrease with the aging process and has been implicated as a possible causative agent in disease states like depression, Alzheimer's and Parkinson's.

Q: Do fibromyalgia sufferers have low methylation problems?
A: Yes, it is possible. Methylation has a kind of seesaw relationship with homocysteine formation and degradation. This means that an increase of homocysteine level in the body is a sure sign of low methylation level and vice versa. Recent scientific evidence indicates that fibromyalgia patients may have high levels of homocysteine.

Q: Why are we only recently hearing about SAM-e? Isn't it just another hype?
A: The main reason is that most of the clinical trials about SAM-e were conducted in Europe, especially Italy. Unlike the United States, European countries are more open to alternative forms of treatment, which have always been practiced in tandem with conventional pharmacological remedies.

Q: Why is it advisable to take only the "enteric-coated" type of SAM-e?
A: Because SAM-e is absorbed mainly through the intestine, using an enteric-coated form allows it to pass intact through the digestive environment of the stomach and be in good shape for absorption when it reaches the small intestine.

Q: Why is it important to store SAM-e properly in a cool and dry environment?
A: Because SAM-e is highly unstable and is easily broken down by heat and moisture.

Q: How does SAM-e actually work in the body?
A: SAM-e's efficacy is due to its versatile chemical nature—that is, its ability to donate its methyl group to acceptor molecules, thereby forming beneficial compounds. The processes in which SAM-e is involved include methylation, transsulfuration and many other lesser-known processes.

Q: How can SAM-e relieve the depressive moods of fibromyalgia patients?
A: By assisting through methylation in the production of several neurotransmitters, which can affect mood-like transforming L-dopa into a mood-regulator called dopamine.

Q: How does SAM-e relieve fatigue symptoms?
A: SAM-e can boost energy levels by assisting in the production of creatine phosphate. Athletes are known to take supplemental forms of creatine phosphate as energy boosters during high-impact sports.

Q: Has it been clinically proven that SAM-e can help fibromyalgia sufferers?
A: Yes, the following have been proven about SAM-e and fibromyalgia in clinical trials:

1. SAM-e was able to improve depressive moods and reduce tender points in fibromyalgia patients.

2. A six-week treatment of fibromyalgia using a daily dose of 800 mg was found to improve symptoms of fatigue, pain, morning stiffness and mood.

3. Another study found that SAM-e was more beneficial than TENS (transcutaneous electrical nerve stimulation) in treating pain and tender points.

Q: Since SAM-e is so expensive, are there any alternative supplements?
A: Yes, another methylation agent is TMG (trimethyl-glycine). The problem is that some scientists believe TMG may not be

involved in the brain cell methylation process and, as such, may not be an exact substitute.

Q: How does SAM-e affect gene abnormality repair, which is regarded as a possible causative factor for fibromyalgia?
A: The probable explanation is that SAM-e, through methylation of DNA and RNA, activates or deactivates genes. Activated genes produce disease-fighting antibodies; deactivated genes regress tumors and cancerous growths. Besides, SAM-e plays an important role in polyamine manufacture. These contain nitrogen that is needed in DNA synthesis and gene expression repairs.

Q: How can SAM-e improve sleep quality for fibromyalgia patients?
A: Through methylation, SAM-e reacts with serotonin to form melatonin. Secreted by the pineal gland, melatonin is responsible for synchronizing hormonal release, thereby regulating the so-called "circadian rhythm," in which daylight promotes melatonin release, while darkness suppresses is.

Q: Why is SAM-e regarded as better and preferable to regular antidepressants?
A: SAM-e has quicker action, with responses as soon as 4 to 7 days. SAM-e leaves no side effects even at very high doses, and will not cause withdrawal reactions if you decide to stop taking it. Besides, unlike antidepressants, it is not a foreign compound in your body, and may, in fact, promote beneficial metabolic processes.

Resources for Help with Fibromyalgia

Information About Fibromyalgia Syndrome

Fibromyalgia Network
P.O. Box 31750
Tucson, AZ 85751-1750
(520) 290-5508 (telephone)
(520) 290-5550 (fax)

American College of Rheumatology
60 Executive Park South, Suite 150
Atlanta, GA 30329
(404) 633-3777

Arthritis Foundation
1330 West Peachtree Street
Atlanta, GA 30309
(404) 872-7100
(800) 283-7800

National Fibromyalgia Research Association Inc.
P.O. Box 500
Salem, OR 97308

Social Security Disability Advocates, Inc.
23930 Michigan Avenue
Dearborn, MI 48124
(800) 628-2887

Social Security and Long Term Disability Insurance Attorney
Scott E. Davis (480) 367-1601
Or e-mail harris.davis@azbar.org

Fibromyalgia Association of Central Texas
2505 Western Drive
Garland, TX 74042-5650
(972) 494-1253

Fibromyalgia Frontiers
Fibromyalgia Association of Greater Washington
13203 Valley Drive
Woodbridge, VA 22191-1531
(703) 790-2324 (telephone)
(703) 494-4103 (fax)

Newsletters about Fibromyalgia

Fibromyalgia Network
Cost: $19
P.O. Box 31750
Tucson, AZ 85751-1750
(520) 290-5508
(800) 853-2929

Fibromyalgia Wellness Letter
Cost: $24.95
P.O. Box 921907
Norcross, GA 30010-1907
(877) 775-0343

Fibromyalgia Times
Cost: $25
P.O. Box 20408
Columbus, OH 43221-0990
(614) 457-4222

Resources for SAM-e

SAM-e can be purchased in most pharmacies, grocery stores, other retail outlets and these importers:

Life Extension Foundation
P.O. Box 229120
Hollywood, FL 33022-9120
(800) 841-5433

Nature Made
(800) 276-2878

Here are some Web sites that were selling SAM-e as of December 12, 1999. Sites are ranked from lowest to highest price.

Price for SAM-e (20 tablets)

Rank	Web Site	Price
1	Immunesupport.com	$17.99
2	Samsstore.com	$18.98
3	Cordette.com	$18.99
4	Drugstore.com	$18.99
5	Mothernature.com	$18.99
6	LEF.org	$25.50
7	Cwinstitute.com	$28.20
8	Iherb.com	$30.00
9	Lifesourcenat.com	$34.99
10	Smart-drugs.com	$36.95
11	Vitanet.com	$37.50
12	Immunonutrition.com	$37.77
13	Vitaminconnection.com	$39.95

Source: www.immunesupport.com/compare.htm

Notes, Recommended Reading and Web Sites

Overview of Fibromyalgia

Adam, N., & Sim, J. (1998). An overview of fibromyalgia syndrome: Mechanisms, differential diagnosis and treatment approaches. *Physiotherapy*, 7(8).

Bennett, R. M. (1999). Emerging concepts in the neurobiology of chronic pain: Evidence of abnormal sensory processing in fibromyalgia. *Mayo Clinic Proceedings*, 74, 385-398.

Bennett, R. M., Campbell, S., Burkhart, C., Clark, S., O'Reilly, C., & Wiens, A. (1991). A multidisciplinary approach to fibromyalgia management. *Journal of Musculoskeletal Medicine*, 8(11), 21-32.

Bennett, R. M., Clark, S. R., Campbell, S. M., & Burkhart, C. S. (1992). Low levels of somatomedin-C in patients with the fibromyalgia syndrome: A possible link between deep sleep and muscle pain. *Arthritis and Rheumatism*, 35 113-116.

Cote, K. A., et al. (1997). Sleep, daytime symptoms, and cognitive performance in patients with fibromyalgia. *Journal of Rheumatology*, 24 (10), 2014-2023.

Dreher, T. (1999). *Fibromyalgia Seminar*. Larkspur, CA: Fibromyalgia Center of Marin.

Goodman, C. C., & Boissannault, G. W. (1998). *Pathology: Implications for the Physical Therapist*. Philadelphia: W.B. Saunders Company.

Hudson, J. I., & Pope, H. G. (1996). The relationship between fibromyalgia and major depressive disorder. *Rheumatic Disease Clinics of North America*, 22(2), 285-303.

Hulme, J. A. (1997). *Fibromyalgia: A handbook for self care and treatment* (2nd ed.). Missoula, MT: Phoenix Publishing Company.

Moldofsky, H. (1998). Sleep, wakefulness, neuroendocrine and immune function in fibromyalgia and chronic fatigue syndrome. Rheumatic Diseases Clinics of North America, 22(2), 219-243.

Russel, I. J. (1998). Fibromyalgia syndrome: Formulating a strategy for relief. *The Journal of Musculoskeletal Medicine*, 15(11), 4-21.

Shaver, J. L., et al. (1997). Sleep, psychological distress, and stress arousal in women with fibromyalgia. *Research in Nursing and Health*, 20(3), 247-257.

Wolfe, H., Smythe, H. A., Yunus, M. B., et al. (1990). The American College of Rheumatology 1990 criteria for the classification of fibromyalgia: Repot of the Multicenter Criteria Committee. *Arthritis and Rheumatism*, 33, 160-172.

Yunus, M., Masi, A. T., Calabro, J. J., Miller, K. A., & Feigenbaum, S. L. (1981). Primary fibromyalgia (fibrositis): Clinical study of 50 patients with matched controls. *Seminars in Arthritis and Rheumatism*, 11, 151-171.

SAM-e and Fibromyalgia

Baldessarini, R. J. (1975). Biological transmethylation involving S-adenosyl-methionine: Development of assay methods and implications for neuropsychiatry. *International Journal of Neurobiology*, 18, 41-67.

Baldessarini, R. J. (1987). Neuropharmacology of S-adenosyl-L-methionine. *American Journal of Medicine*, 83 (suppl. 5A), 95-103.

Berger, R., & Nowak, H. (1987). A new medical approach to the treatment of osteoarthritis: Report of an open phase IV study with ademetionine (gumbaral). *American Journal of Medicine*, 83(suppl. 5A), 84-88.

Cantoni, G. L. (1953). S-adenosylmethionine: A new intermediate formed enzymatically from L-methionine and adenosine-triphosphate. *Journal of Biological Chemistry*, 204, 403-416.

Chiang, P. K., Gordon, R. K., Tal, J., et al. (1996). S-adenosylmethionine and methylation. *Federation of The American Society of Experimental Biology Journal*, 10, 471-480.

Clouatre, D. (1999). *All about SAM-e*. New York: Avery Publishing Group.

Cooney, C., & Lawren, B. (1999). *Methyl Magic*. Kansas City: Andrew McMeel Books.

DiBenedetto, P., Iona, L. G., & Zidarich, V. (1993). Clinical evaluation of S-adenosyl-O-methionine versus transcutaneous electrical nerve stimulation in primary fibromyalgia. *Current Therapeutic Research*, 53, 222-229.

Friedel, H. A., Goa, L. L., & Benfield, P. (1989). S-adenosyl-L-methionine. *Drugs*, 38, 3889-3917.

Gatto, C., et al. (1985). Analgesizing effect of a methyl donor (S-adenosyl methionine) in migraine: An open clinical trial. *International Journal of Clinical Pharmacology Research*, 5, 39-49.

Grassetto, M., & Varotto, A. (1995). Primary fibromyalgia is responsive to S-adenosyl-L-methionine. *Current Therapeutic Research*, 55, 797-806.

Grazi, S., & Costa, M. (1999). *The European Arthritis and Depression Breakthrough! SAM-e*. Rocklin, CA: Prima Health.

Guibidori, P., Galli-Kienle, J., Catto, E., & Stramentindi, G. (1984). Transmethylation, transsulfuration and aminopropylation reactions of S-adenosyl-L-methionine in vivo. *Journal of Biological Chemistry*, 259, 4205-4211.

Jacobsen, S., Danneskiold-Samsoe, B., Anderson, R. B. (1991). Oral S-adenosylmethionine in primary fibromyalgia: Double blind clinical evaluation. *Scandinavian Journal of Rheumatology*, 20(4), 294-302.

Mitchell, D. (1999). *The SAM-e Solution*. New York: Warner Books Inc.

Murray, M., & Pizzorno, J. (1998). *Encyclopedia of Natural Medicine* (2nd ed.). Rocklin, CA: Prima Health.

Osman, E., et al. (1993). Review article: S-adenosyl-L-methionine–a new therapeutic agent in liver disease? *Alimentary Pharmacology and Therapeutics*, 1, 21-28.

Salvatore, F., Borek, E., Zappia, V., et al. (1977). *The Biochemistry of Adenosyl-Methionine*. New York: Columbia University Press.

Stramentinoli, G. (1987). Pharmacological aspects of S-adenosylmethionine: Pharmacokinetics and pharmacodynamics. *American Journal of Medicine*, 83(suppl. 5A), 35-42.

Tavoni, A., Vitalie, C., Benbardier, S., & Pasero, G. (1987). Evaluation of S-adenosylmethionine in primary fibromyalgia: A double-blind crossover study. *American Journal of Medicine,* 88(5A), 107-110.

Volkman, H., Norregaard, J., Jacobson, S., et al. (1997). D-blind, placebo-controlled crossover study of intravenous S-adenosyl-L-methionine in patients with fibromyalgia. *Scandinavian Journal of Rheumatology,* 26(3), 206-211.

Fibromyalgia Medications and Their Problems: How to Come off Them

Breggin, P. R. & Cohen, D. (1999). *Your Drug May Be Your Problem.* Reading, MA: Perseus Books.

Garner, E. M., Kelly, M. W., Thompson, D. F. (1993). Tricyclic antidepressant withdrawal syndrome. *Annals of Pharmacotherapy,* 27, 1068-1072.

Johnson, J. A. & Bootman, J. L. (1995). Drug-related morbidity and mortality: A cost-of-illness model. *Archives of Internal Medicine,* 155, 1949-1956.

Lazarou, J., Pomeranz, B. H. & Corey, P. N. (1998). Incidence of adverse drug reactions in hospitalized patients: A meta-analysis of prospective studies. *Journal of the American Medical Association,* 279, 1200-1205.

Manasse, H. R. Jr. (1989). Medication use in an imperfect world: Drug misadventuring as an issue of public policy. Part I. *American Journal of Hospital Pharmacy,* 46, 929-944.

Manasse, H. R. Jr. (1989). Medication use in an imperfect world: Drug misadventuring as an issue of public policy. Part II. *American Journal of Hospital Pharmacy,* 46, 1141-1152.

Maxmen, J. S. & Ward, N. G. (1995). *Psychotropic Drugs: Fast Facts* (2nd). New York: W. W. Norton and Company.

The Merk Manual of Medical Information (home ed.). (1997). Whitehouse Station, NJ: Merck & Co., Inc.

Mindell, E. L. & Hopkins, V. (1999). *Prescription Alternatives.* Los Angeles: Keats Publishing.

The USP Guide to Medicines (1st). (1996). New York: Avon Books.

Wolf, R. M. (1997). Anti-depressant withdrawal reactions. *American Family Physician, 56,* 455-462.

Other Drug-Free Fibromyalgia Relief and Self-Care Strategies

Abraham, G. (1992). Management of fibromyalgia: Rationale for the use of magnesium and malic acid. *Journal of Nutritional Medicine,* 3, 49-59.

Balch, J. F. & Balch, P. A. (1998). *A To Z Guide to Supplements.* New York: Avery Publishing Group.

Berkson, B. (1998). *All About B Vitamins.* New York: Avery Publishing Group.

Butler, G. & Hope, T. (1945). *Managing Your Mind.* New York: Oxford University Press.

Kisner, C. & Colby, L. A. (1985). *Therapeutic Exercise: Foundations and Techniques.* Philadelphia: F. A. Davis Company.

Netzers, C. T. (1999). *Big Book of Miracle Cures.* New York: Dell Publishing.

Passwater, R. A. (1998). *All About Antioxidants.* New York: Avery Publishing Group.

US Dept. of Agriculture; US Dept. of Health and Human Services. (1995). *Nutrition and your health: Dietary guidelines for Americans* – E-text (4th). Washington, DC: Author.

Woodham, A. & Peters, D. (1997). *Encyclopedia of Healing Therapies.* New York: DK Publishing Inc.

Fibromyalgia Disability Issues

Burkhart, C. S., Sharon, R. C. & Bennett, R. M. (1991). The fibromyalgia impact questionnaire: Development and validation. *Journal of Rheumatology,* 18, 728-733.

Cathney, M. A., Wolfe, F. & Klienkeksel, S. M. (1998). Functional ability and work status in patients with fibromyalgia. *Arthritis Care,* 1, 85-98.

Mason, J. H., Simms, R. W., Goldenberg, D. L., et al. (1989). The impact of fibromyalgia on work: A comparison to rheumatoid arthritis. *Arthritis and Rheumatism,* 32, R7.

Potter, W. J. (1992). Helping fibromyalgia patients obtain Social Security benefits. *Journal of Musculoskeletal Medicine,* 9(9), 65-74.

Silverman, S. L. & Mason, J. H. (1992). Measuring the functional impact of fibromyalgia. *Journal of Musculoskeletal Medicine,* 9(7), 15-24.

Social Security Administration. (1986). Social Security regulations: Rules for determining disability and blindness. Washington, DC: U.S. Dept. of Health and Human Services. Social Security Administration. Office of Disability, SSA Publication No. 64-014.

Some Fibromyalgia Research Websites

www.lef.org

www.immunesupport.com/fms_research

www.myalgia.com

www.nih.gov/niams/healthinfo

www.cbshealthwatch.aol.com

www.sleepfoundation.org

www.healthology.com

www.niddk.nih.gov/health

www.hsc.missouri.edu

www.fmnetnews.com

Glossary

Acetylcholine (ACh). The chemical transmitter of the nerve impulse across a synapse. It is also released from endings of parasympathetic nerves (cholinergic nerves) upon stimulation. Some of its actions include cardiac slowing, dilation of arteries, increased gastrointestinal activity.

Adenosine triphosphate (ATP). The body's main energy molecule.

Akathesia (restless legs). A condition that often occurs just before falling asleep. Usually occurs in people under stress, it is characterized by spontaneous, uncontrollable leg movements.

Alzheimer's disease. A disease of the brain that is characterized by a progressive diminishing of cognitive functions, especially in areas of short-term memory.

Amino acid. Organic acid containing one or more amino groups (NH_2) and a carboxyl group (CO_2H). These form the essential component of proteins.

Aminopropylation. The process in which SAM-e donates a methyl group to produce spermidine and spermine. These substances are necessary for cell growth, differentiation, nerve tissue repair, etc.

Anti-anxiety drugs. Drugs used to treat states of worry and anxiety.

Antidepressant. Any agent used in treating pathologic depressive states.

Anti-inflammatory. Any agent that reduces an inflammatory response and associated pain and swelling.

Antioxidant. A substance that prevents oxidation. An example is glutathione.

Atom. The smallest unit of an element. Atoms aggregate to form molecules.

Auto-antibody. Antibody that is produced in and reacts with a person's own antigen.

Auto-immune disease. Any disease characterized by injury to the tissue caused by an apparent immunologic reaction of the host with his own tissues. This is different from autoimmune response, with which it may or may not be associated.

Biopsy. The removal and examination of tissue from the living body for the purpose of diagnosis.

Catecholamine. An amine compound derived from catechol, such as epinephrine and norepinephrine, which are involved with nervous transmission, vascular tone and other metabolic activities.

Chronic fatigue syndrome (CFS). A condition that is characterized by extreme and continuous fatigue.

Circadian rhythm. Denoting the rhythm of biologic phenomena that cycle approximately every 24 hours. Example: Cortisol secretion rises in the early-morning hours, peaks by the time we awake, and falls in the evening.

Cirrhosis. A liver disease that is irreversible. Liver tissues are damaged by agents such as alcohol, viruses and toxins.

CoEnzyme. A nonprotein organic compound produced by living cells, which plays an important role in the activation of enzymes, e.g., riboflavin.

Cofactor. A substance whose presence is required to bring about the action of an enzyme.

Controlled study. A study in which one group of subjects is used as a basis of comparison with another group. The subjects are also called controls.

Cortisol. A steroid hormone that is isolated from the adrenal cortex. It provides resistance to stresses and maintains a number of enzyme systems. Also called hydrocortisone.

Cysteine. Amino acid that contains sulfur.

Deconditioning. This usually occurs in people with sedentary lifestyles or people who have been inactive and on bed rest for a long time. Some deconditioning effects include decreased cardiac output, vital capacity, work capacity, etc.

Delta sleep. The deep phase of the sleep cycle. This is also known as the restorative phase of sleep, in which brain wave activity is described as "delta wave."

Demethylation. Removal of a methyl group from any molecule, such as DNA.

Deoxyribonucleic acid (DNA). The molecular basis of genetics. Responsible for gene expression.

Detoxification. Removal of toxins from the body.

Dopamine. A neurotransmitter produced in the brain. Produced by methylation of L-dopa. Dopamine is a principal mood regulator.

Double-blind study. A study in which two types of interventions are compared, and neither the study participants nor the investigators (thus, double) know what the intervention is. The participants are not influenced by knowledge about the intervention.

DSHEA. Also called Dietary Supplement Health and Education Act, passed by Congress in 1994. This act allows drug manufacturers to produce and market any supplement with a good safety record without an FDA prior authorization, as long as these companies do not make any outrageous claims about the efficacy of the supplements.

Enteric-coated. A term used to describe the layer applied to a tablet or capsule that protects the tablet's or capsule's contents from digestion by the stomach environment, thus allowing the contents to get to the intestinal tract.

Enzyme. A protein molecule that is able to increase the rate of chemical reactions.

Fibro-fog. A memory and concentration impairment of fibromyalgia patients.

Fibromyalgia. A chronic disorder characterized by persistent and widespread muscle soreness, stiffness, chronic fatigue and many other symptoms, markedly including well-defined painful spots called "tender points."

Fibromyalgia Impact Questionnaire. A self-administered functional outcome test for fibromyalgia patients in areas of depression, functional and work capacity, anxiety, sleep, pain, stiffness, fatigue and general well-being.

Fibrositis. A former name for fibromyalgia, it is the inflammation of fibrous or connective tissue of the muscles. As we now know, there is no inflammatory process in fibromyalgia.

Free radical. An atom or molecule with an unpaired electron that can trigger a series of oxidative reactions. They can damage beneficial systems like proteins, fats, membranes, cells, etc.

Glutathione. The body's powerful antioxidant. It also detoxifies the liver. Glutathione seeks out toxins, attaches to them, and thereby makes them water soluble and able to be eliminated in the urine.

Histamine. An amine that can cause bronchiolar constriction, arteriolar dilatation, increased gastric secretion and a fall in blood pressure.

Homocysteine. A toxic amino acid that is a by-product of methionine metabolism.

Integrative medicine. A health care practice that addresses human problems in all of their physical, psychological and spiritual ramifications. It uses all available treatment techniques, which it integrates to treat the human person.

Inflammation. A tissue reaction to irritation, infection or injury, characterized by localized heat, swelling, redness, and pain, that can result in some loss of function.

Irritable bowel syndrome (IBS). A chronic condition characterized by abdominal pain, stomach upset, constipation or diarrhea.

Juvenile primary fibromyalgia. Fibromyalgia that affects children and has no associated conditions.

Libido. Emotional and instinctual energies and desires, usually referring to the sexual instinct.

Lipids. A chemical name for fats and oils.

Lupus. A disease that is characterized by joint pain, fatigue, muscle soreness and skin rashes. There is also joint swelling and organ disease like blood in the urine. Laboratory study would indicate elevated blood sedimentation rates, depressed white blood cell count and increased anti-DNA antibodies.

Lyme disease. A disease caused by the *Borrelia burgdorferi* bacteria transmitted by deer ticks. Symptoms begin as a large red spot on the thigh or buttocks, trunk or armpit that expands to about 6 inches in diameter. Other symptoms include fatigue, fever, headaches, muscle pain and joint pain.

Melatonin. A hormone that is produced in the pineal gland with the assistance of SAM-e. It is responsible for regulating the sleep-wake cycle.

Metabolic pathway. A step-by-step order in which biochemical processes take place in the body.

Metabolism. The biochemical processes in the body that sustain life, for example include fat metabolism.

Metabolites. Harmful by-products of metabolism, like lactic acid produced during muscle action.

Methionine. An essential amino acid that is the building block for SAM-e and homocysteine manufacture.

Methyl donor. Any substance that has the ability to lose its methyl group to another substance.

Methyl group. A reactive unit of organic chemical compound, containing one carbon and three hydrogen atoms. It changes the nature of whatever molecule it gets attached to. For example, when attached to a section of DNA, it prevents any damages to the genetic code.

Methylation. The process in which SAM-e loses its methyl group to another acceptor molecule.

Migraine. A recurrent, intense headache, usually localized on one side of the head and characterized by nausea, vomiting and visual disturbances.

Muscle spasms. Uncontrollable muscle activity.

Myofascial pain syndrome. A painful condition of skeletal muscles, characterized by one or several painful sites or trigger points located within muscles or tendons. When these sites are stimulated by palpation, they produce pain in the area of the patient's symptoms.

Neurotransmitters. Chemical substances often referred to as chemical messengers. They are released from nerve cells to activate receptor sites in other nerve cells, and thereby propagate nerve impulses. Examples are dopamine and norepinephrine.

NSAID. This stands for non-steroidal anti-inflammatory drug. These drugs are often prescribed to relieve pain by reducing inflammation.

Osteoarthritis. A degenerative joint disease characterized by degeneration of articular cartilage and hypertrophy of bone, accompanied by pain. Pain increases with activity and subsides with rest.

Oxidation. A chemical process in which electrons from one reactant (reducing agent) are transferred to another (oxidizing agent).

Palpitation. A rapid or forceful heartbeat, which the patient feels.

Phosphocreatine. A creatine phosphoric acid compound, a major source of energy in muscle contraction.

Polymyalgia rheumatica. A condition characterized by severe pain and stiffness in the neck and in the muscles of shoulders and hips. It can be accompanied by another condition called temporal (giant cell) arteritis.

Private disability insurance. A nongovernmental and privately sponsored insurance program that pays benefits to its customers who become unable to work.

Protein. A complex nitrogenous substance of high molecular weight that contains fundamental structural units known as amino acids. Protein is present in the cells of all animals and plants, and is intimately involved in all phases of chemical and physical activity of the cell.

Proteoglycan. A complex of polysaccharide and protein, present in structural tissues of vertebrates like bone, and also in cell surfaces.

Prozac (fluoxetine). An SSRI drug whose main function is to increase the levels of serotonin in the body. Used to treat depression.

PTSD (Post-traumatic stress disorder). This is an anxiety disorder caused by the experience of an overwhelming traumatic event which a person later experiences repeatedly.

Rapid eye movements (REM). A sleep phase characterized by rapid eye movements and high brain electrical activity, somewhat like that of an awake state.

Reynaud's phenomenon. A condition in which the small blood vessels constrict, thereby decreasing blood flow to the extremities. The fingers turn very white on exposure to cold.

Rheumatoid arthritis. An autoimmune condition characterized by symmetrical inflammation of joints, usually in the hands and feet.

Serotonin. A central nervous system neurotransmitter. Can also be released by blood platelets following injury. Serotonin plays a role in mood regulation.

Sjögren's Syndrome. A condition characterized by a distinctive type of dry mouth and dry eyes. There may be oral and swallowing problems. It is an autoimmune condition associated with arthritis, muscle inflammation, thyroid and kidney problems.

Sleep spindles. A sleep phase in which brain activity diminishes to occasional spikes.

Somatomedin. A peptide present in plasma, formed in the liver or kidney. It can stimulate synthesis of protein, RNA or DNA.

SSA (Social Security Administration). A government agency that administers government-sponsored welfare programs.

SSDI (Social Security Disability Insurance). A disability insurance program sponsored by the Social Security Administration for those who have worked for at least 5 years before becoming disabled.

SSI (Supplementary Security Income). A government-sponsored disability insurance program for workers. Similar to SSDI in eligibility criteria, but different in the financial qualification requirement.

SSRI (selective serotonin reuptake inhibitors). A group of antidepressants that act by decreasing levels of serotonin in the brain. Example: Prozac.

Substance P. A polypeptide found in the brain, especially the substantia nigra. It is a sensory transmitter that mediates pain perception.

Syndrome. A complex condition, often with other associated conditions.

Tender points. Well-defined painful spots on the body.

Tension headache. A type of headache characterized by pain around the head and neck regions.

TMG (trimethyl-glycine). Also known as "betaine." A methylated version of glycine. Another efficient methyl donor.

TMJ (temporomandibular joint). Fibromyalgia patients sometimes complain of pain in this jaw region, which can radiate to other parts of the face.

Transmethylation. A process in which there is a transfer of methyl groups between methyl donors and methyl acceptors.

Transsulfuration. A process in which homocysteine loses its sulfur to produce the amino acids cysteine, taurine or cystathionine.

Uncontrolled study. A research study in which investigators and subjects are aware of the intervention being administered.

Whiplash injury. A neck injury caused by the sudden jerking of the head forward and backward.

Withdrawal symptoms. The unpleasant effects of stopping the ingestion of an addictive chemical substance.

Index

A

Abnormal brain function, 21, 55
Acetyl L-carnitine, 135-136
Activity level, 95
Adapin. *See* Doxepin and
  Tricyclics.
Addiction
  physiological, 33
  psychological, 32
  See also Dependence.
Addictive medications
  how to come off, 71, 73-75
  withdrawal reactions and, 75
Adenosine triphosphate (ATP), 22
  defined, 163
Aerobics
  body sculpting, 116
  examples of, 114
  funk, 116
  high impact, 115
  low impact, 115
Aggressive behaviors, 36
Allergens, 59
Alpha-EEG anomaly, 13
  See also Sleep disorders
Alprazolam (Xanax), 27
Alternative medicine, xiv
Alzheimer's, 64
American Association of Chronic
  Fatigue Syndrome
  Conference, 56
American College of
  Rheumatology, 3
*American Journal of Hospital
  Pharmacy*, 31

Aminopropylation, 52-53
Amitriptyline (Elavil), xii, 26
Anafranil. *See* Clomipramine
  and Tricyclics.
Anger, 91-92
Anticholinergic effects, 34
Antidepressants, adverse effects of,
  34-40
Anxiolytics, 27
  adverse effects of, 37
Aromatherapy, 90
Associated fibromyalgia
  symptoms, 7
Ativan. *See* Lorazepam and
  Benzodiazepines.
ATP. *See* Adenosine triphosphate
  (ATP).
Autoimmune disease
  defined, 172
  disorders, 22
  fibromyalgia and, 7
  SAM-e and, 55

B

Benzodiazepines
  examples of short and
  long acting, 27
Bile salts, 63
Borrelio burgdorferi, 8
  See Lyme disease.
Breathing exercise, 82-84
  diaphragmatic, 83
Breggin (Dr.), xii
Brown, Richard (Dr.), 57

Order Form

I would like to order additional copies of
Fibromyalgia Relief: The SAM-e Solution

1–24 copies	$14.95 each
25-99 copies (40% discount)	$8.97 each
100-499 copies (45% discount).	$8.22 each
500-999 copies (50% discount).	$7.47 each
1000-2499 copies (55% discount)	$6.73 each
2500-4999 copies (60% discount)	$5.98 each
5000-9999 copies (70% discount)	$4.49 each
10,000+ copies	negotiable

Shipping & Handling:
. . . . . 1st copy $3.50, each additional copy $.55

No. copies _____ x Price each $_____ = $_____

Shipping & Handling ($3.50 + $.55 x _____) = $_____

Grand Total = $_____

Name _____

Street _____

City/State/Zip _____

Please send check or money order to:

PTS Publishing Company
P.O. Box 663
Old Bridge, NJ 08857

(732) 296-1111

Notes

Notes

Notes

Notes